AF774682

Cornelis J. P. Thijn

Arthrography of the Knee Joint

Foreword by J. R. Blickman

With 173 Figures
(209 Separate Illustrations)

Springer-Verlag
Berlin Heidelberg New York 1979

Dr. CORNELIS JACOB PIETER THIJN
Department of Radiology, State University Hospital
Groningen (Netherlands)

ISBN-13: 978-3-642-46400-3 e-ISBN-13: 978-3-642-46398-3
DOI: 10.1007/978-3-642-46398-3

Library of Congress Cataloging in Publication Data. Thijn, Cornelis Jacob Pieter, 1933 – Arthrography of the knee joint. Bibliography: p. Includes index. 1. Knee-Diseases-Diagnosis. 2. Knee-Radiography. 3. Contrast media. I. Title. RC951.T47 617'.582 78-31982

This work is subject to copyright. All rights are reserved, whether the whole or part of the material is concerned, specifically those of translation, reprinting, re-use of illustrations, broadcasting, reproduction by photocopying machine or similar means, and storage in data banks.

Under § 54 of the German Copyright Law, where copies are made for other than private use, a fee is payable to the publisher, the amount of the fee to be determined by agreement with the publisher.

© by Springer-Verlag Berlin Heidelberg 1979
Softcover reprint of the hardcover 1st edition 1979

The use of registered names, trademarks, etc. in this publication does not imply, even in the absence of a specific statement, that such names are exempt from the relevant protective laws and regulations and therefore free for general use.

Reproduction of figures: Gustav Dreher GmbH, Stuttgart

2180/3130-543210

Foreword

It is a great pleasure to introduce this book and its writer to the reader. Dr. Thijn has been interested in double contrast studies since he wrote his thesis on the double contrast examination of the colon. It would sound facetious to state that after he exhausted this field, he was in need of some other area where the same technique could be used. However, in the same exact and thorough way as in his colon studies, he has examined the knee joint.

Considering that the knee is one of the most heavily taxed joints in man, with a multitude of afflictions, many of them closely connected with the age of the individual, radiological investigation has shown very few innovations over the decades. The true anteroposterior and lateral projections were – and still are – the mainstay of the investigation. Projections of the intercondylar fossa, and true patellar projections were used incidentally.

Just prior to World War II the advent of arthrography as a double contrast investigation, as promoted by Oberholzer, was a real breakthrough.

Many papers can be cited that propagate single contrast studies either by gaseous or by positive contrast agents. But through the years double contrast studies slowly attracted more attention as the method of choice. Dr. Thijn's studies add two important values to the arthrographic literature on the inner anatomy of the knee joint: firstly, he collaborated closely with the orthopedic department of the Groningen University Hospital, and especially with Dr. Eikelaar, one of the promotors of arthroscopy. A systematic study using both double contrast arthrography and arthroscopy methods in a critical way is the backbone of this book.

Secondly, the book's value is increased tremendously by its detailed study of the roentgen anatomy of knee structures other than meniscus or joint capsule. The information on the cruciate ligaments, Hoffa body, and – mainly – on the joint cartilage has furthered our knowledge to a great extent.

May this book be of value to the many doctors that have been entrusted with the primary task of keeping people on their feet.

State University Groningen — Prof. Dr. J.R. Blickman

Preface

Arthrography of the knee joint is not a new method of examination. General and orthopedic surgeons have been making use of arthrographic results for decades.
The majority of radiologists who apply this method focus solely on the presence or absence of meniscal lesions. Not only is this regrettable, but it also implies an underevaluation of arthrography. With an optimal arthrographic technique, not only meniscal lesions, but also patellar chondropathy, cruciate ligament ruptures, and degenerative lesions of the articular cartilage can be diagnosed.
With the exception of the diagnosis of cruciate ligament ruptures, double contrast arthrography is the best variant of all arthrographic techniques.
Each of the above mentioned lesions will receive ample attention in the various chapters. Whenever necessary, the anatomy is discussed in direct relation to the structures and lesions to be demonstrated, thus making each chapter a comprehensive entity. In addition, an impression will be given of the correlation between double contrast arthrography and arthroscopy.
It should be stressed once again that a positive correlation can be ensured only if optimal technical execution of the examination is combined with evaluation by an experienced radiodiagnostician.

Groningen, February 1979 C.J.P. THIJN

Contents

1	History of Arthrography	1
2	Technique of Double Contrast Arthrography	3
2.1	Introduction	3
2.2	Injection of Contrast Media	4
2.3	Arthrography	6
2.3.1	Cruciate Ligaments	6
2.3.2	Menisci	6
2.3.3	Patellofemoral Joint	9
2.3.3.1	Lateral Projections	9
2.3.3.2	Tangential Projections	9
2.4	Aftercare and Complications of Arthrography	10
2.4.1	Hydrops	11
2.4.2	Allergic Reactions	12
2.4.3	Air Embolism	12
2.4.4	Arthritis	12
3	Meniscal Lesions	13
3.1	Specific Anatomy	13
3.1.1	Medial Meniscus	13
3.1.2	Lateral Meniscus	15
3.2	Meniscal Functions	16
3.3	Friction and Lubrication	17
3.3.1	Interface Lubrication	17
3.3.2	Buffer Lubrication	17
3.3.3	Elastohydrodynamic Lubrication	17
3.3.4	Sponge Lubrication	18
3.3.5	Lubrication by a Transient Increase in Viscosity	18
3.4	Etiology of Meniscal Lesions	18
3.4.1	Mobility of the Menisci	18
3.4.2	Risk-Increasing Factors	19
3.5	Normal Radiologic Anatomy of the Menisci	20
3.5.1	Medial Meniscus	20
3.5.2	Normal Lateral Meniscus	25
3.5.3	Spurious Meniscal Lesions	27
3.6	Meniscal Lesions	32
3.6.1	Meniscal Ruptures	32
3.6.1.1	Tangential Incisure	32

3.6.1.2 Longitudinal Ruptures 36
3.6.1.3 Fish Mouth Ruptures 40
3.6.1.4 Transverse Ruptures 40
3.6.1.5 Combined Ruptures 41
3.6.2 Types of Discoid Meniscus 43
3.6.3 Degeneration of Meniscal Cartilage 46
3.6.3.1 Primary Degeneration 46
3.6.3.2 Secondary Degeneration 50
3.6.4 State After Meniscectomy 52
3.7 Correlation Between Arthrography and Arthroscopy . . . 55

4 Lesions of the Patellofemoral Joint 61

4.1 Anatomy and Physiology of the Patellofemoral Joint . . . 61
4.2 Articular Cartilage 64
4.2.1 Histology 64
4.2.2 Nutrition of Cartilage 65
4.2.3 Properties of Cartilage 65
4.2.4 Cartilage Degeneration 66
4.2.5 Normal Radiologic Anatomy 67
4.3. Etiology of Patellar Chondropathy 72
4.3.1 General Aspects 72
4.3.2 Mechanical Lesions of the Patellar Cartilage 73
4.3.2.1 Exogenous Factors 73
Direct Lesion of the Patella 73
Overstress 75
Fractures 75
4.3.2.2 Endogenous Factors 75
Patellar Dysplasia 75
Patella Partita 78
Dysplasia of the Facies Patellaris Femoris 78
High Patella 82
Low Patella 83
Increased Patellar Mobility 83
Increased Pressure in the Patellofemoral Joint 85
4.3.3 Non-Mechanical Lesions of the Patellar Cartilage 85
4.4 Radiologic Diagnosis of Patellar Chondropathy 87
4.4.1 Radiologic Examination Without Contrast Medium . . . 87
4.4.2 Double Contrast Arthrography 89
4.5 Correlation Between Double Contrast Arthrography and Arthroscopy 93

5 Cruciate Ligaments 97

5.1 Anatomy of the Cruciate Ligaments 97
5.2 Radiologic Technique 100
5.3 Radiologic Anatomy of the Cruciate Ligaments 102
5.3.1 Anterior Cruciate Ligament 102
5.3.2 Posterior Cruciate Ligament 105

5.4 Etiology of Cruciate Ligament Ruptures 107
5.5 Cruciate Ligament Pathology 108
5.5.1 Abnormal Delimitation of the Cruciate Ligaments 109
5.5.2 Abnormal Displacement of the Tibia in Relation to the Femur 113
5.5.3 Irregular Structures Within the Cruciate Ligament Compartments 116
5.6 Accuracy of Arthrographic Cruciate Ligament Diagnosis . 117

6 Joint Capsule, Collateral Ligaments, Hoffa Body and Bursae 119
6.1 Capsule, Hoffa Body, and Collateral Ligaments 119
6.2 Bursae 126
6.2.1 Suprapatellar Bursa 127
6.2.2 Semimembranosogastrocnemial Bursa 128
6.2.3 Popliteal Bursa 134

7 Lesions of the Articular Cartilage 135
7.1 General Aspects 135
7.2 Etiology and Double Contrast Arthrography 135
7.2.1 Primary Form 136
7.2.2 Secondary Form 136
7.2.2.1 Direct Injury 136
7.2.2.2 Indirect Injury 137
Meniscal Lesions 137
Cruciate and Collateral Ligament Lesions 140
Osteochondritis Dissecans 140
Inflammations 140
Changed Pressures 140
Hemophilia 140
Metabolic Disorders 141

References 145

Subject Index 153

1 History of Arthrography

The first arthrograms of the knee were taken by Robinson and Werndorff in 1905, after oxygen insufflation into the knee joint. Arthrography with the aid of gas as a negative contrast medium remained the sole method in use for several decades. The joint work of Bircher and Oberholzer (1934), who studied 700 arthrograms taken by the negative contrast method, demonstrated the value of this technique in the diagnosis of "dérangement interne". Arthrography of details under fluoroscopic control was an important advance. Wiener (1967) reports that negative contrast arthrography was the method most widely used in the United States until recently. A disadvantage of negative contrast arthrography lies in the uncomfortable swelling of the joint as a result of gas insufflation. The risk of air embolism is small, although some instances have been described (Bircher, 1933; Kleinberg, 1927).

Michaelis (1931) was the first to use a positive contrast medium in arthrography. He used Uroselectan, and subsequently other agents such as Diodone, Perabrodil, and Umbradil were also used. The agents initially used caused marked irritation of the synovium, and pain (Boyd, 1934). The introduction of less irritant contrast media of course led to a reduction of untoward side effects. Contrast media such as Hypaque (Wiener, 1967), Conray (Jelaso, 1968), Renografin (Kiss and Moir, 1968), and Urografin have since been used on a large scale. Mention should be made of the studies of Fischedick (1960a, b, 1963, 1969a) and Ficat (1957, 1962, 1970a, b), who are advocates of positive contrast arthrography. Roebuck (1977) prefers Dimer X as the ideal contrast medium.

In addition to negative and positive contrast arthrography, double contrast arthrography evolved. Bircher (1931) was the first to use this technique. The complications caused by the positive contrast medium initially precluded worldwide use of this method, but when less irritating contrast media became available, Lindblom (1948) gave strong impetus to a wider use of double contrast arthrography. Further improvements were introduced by Van de Berg and Crèvecoeur (1951, 1953, 1955). Andren and Wehlin (1960) used no more than 20–50 ml gas beside the positive contrast medium, and this significantly reduced the untoward complications. Leroux (1960) was unable to demonstrate a difference between the results obtained with double contrast arthrography and those of positive contrast arthrography. Freiberger et al. (1966), using the double contrast method advocated by Andren and Wehlin, demonstrated a positive correlation between the arthrographic and the operative findings in 91% of their patients. The monograph written by Ricklin, Rüttimann and Del Buono (1964, 1971) contributed much to a more extensive use of double contrast arthrography. Good results have since been obtained with this method by Butt et al. (1969), Nicholas (1970), Staple (1972), Angell (1971), Hall (1976), and Thijn (1968, 1971, 1974, 1976).

2 Technique of Double Contrast Arthrography

2.1 Introduction

Negative contrast arthrography after insufflation of air, oxygen, or some other gas is obsolete. The differences in radiolucency between the internal structures of the knee and the gas introduced are too small to permit detection of minor changes such as small meniscal ruptures and cartilage degenerations. Positive contrast arthrography produces good results in demonstrating meniscal lesions. More superficial cartilaginous lesions, such as patellar chondropathy and degenerative lesions of other articular cartilage, disappear under a covering layer of contrast medium in this technique. Double contrast arthrography is more suitable for demonstration of superficial cartilaginous lesions because the internal structures of the knee are covered by only a thin layer of contrast medium, and thus contrast against the air introduced (Fig. 1).

This chapter describes only the technique of double contrast arthrography and, in the interest of a general survey, explains the entire procedure. The results of double contrast arthrography as compared with arthroscopic and operative findings will be discussed in the specific sections.

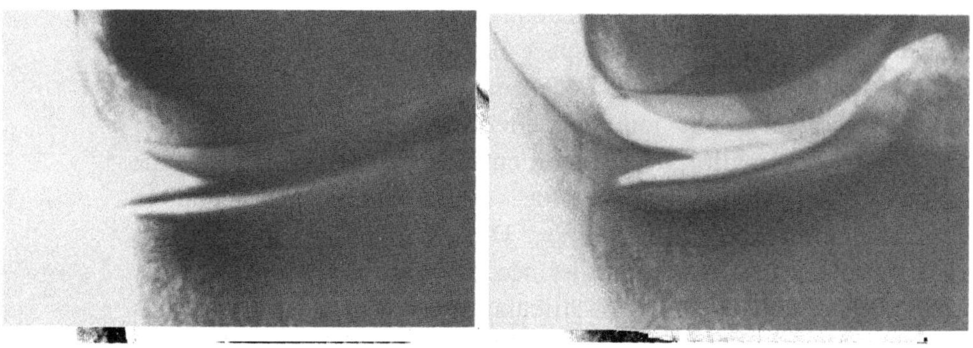

Fig. 1. Single contrast and double contrast arthrography of the medial meniscus in the same patient

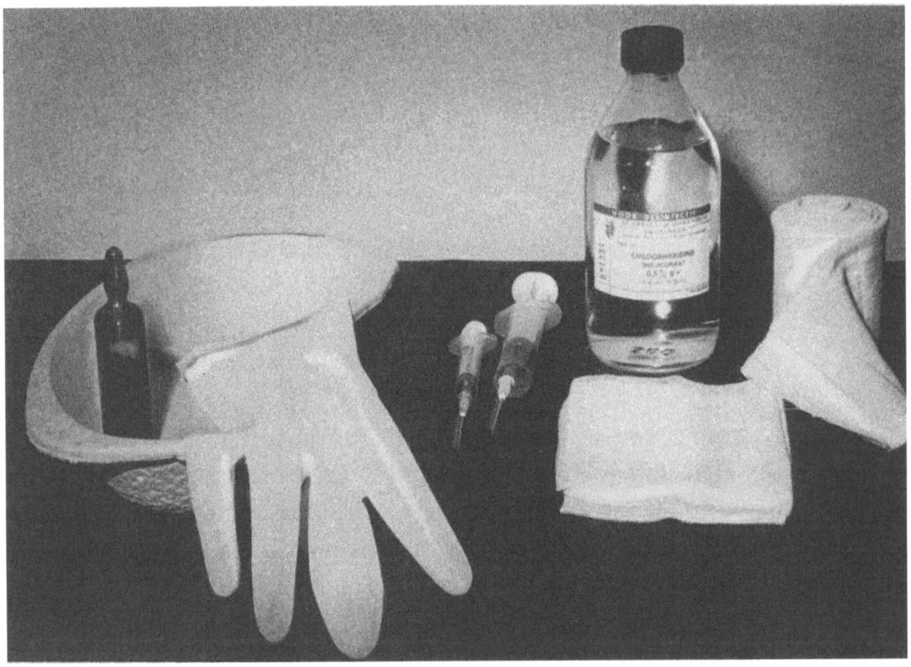

Fig. 2. Equipment required for double contrast arthrography

2.2 Injection of Contrast Media

The patient lies on the table with the knee supported by a triangular cushion. The exterior of the knee is carefully disinfected (Fig. 2). Starting at the injection site, 1 cm dorsal to the lateral margin of the patella and at half the height of the patella, a piece of gauze soaked in tincture of iodine or some other good disinfectant is moved in a spiral pattern over the skin (Fig. 3). Repetition of this procedure is imperative. The investigator should wear sterile gloves. With the knee joint entirely relaxed, the radiologist moves the patella as far laterally as possible, thus slightly enlarging the space between the patellar cartilage and the femoral condyle. Local anesthesia of the injection site is unnecessary. The joint is punctured with a thin needle of about 4 cm length, placed on an empty 2 ml syringe. The needle is inserted parallel to the table surface and perpendicular to the longitudinal axis of the leg. During puncture, the capsule, which is felt as a slight resistance, is passed; the needle must now have entered the intra-articular space. The lateral displacement of the patella can now be abolished, and the fingers of the left hand from now on keep the needle fixed in an absolutely unchanging position. Synovia is regularly sucked into the empty

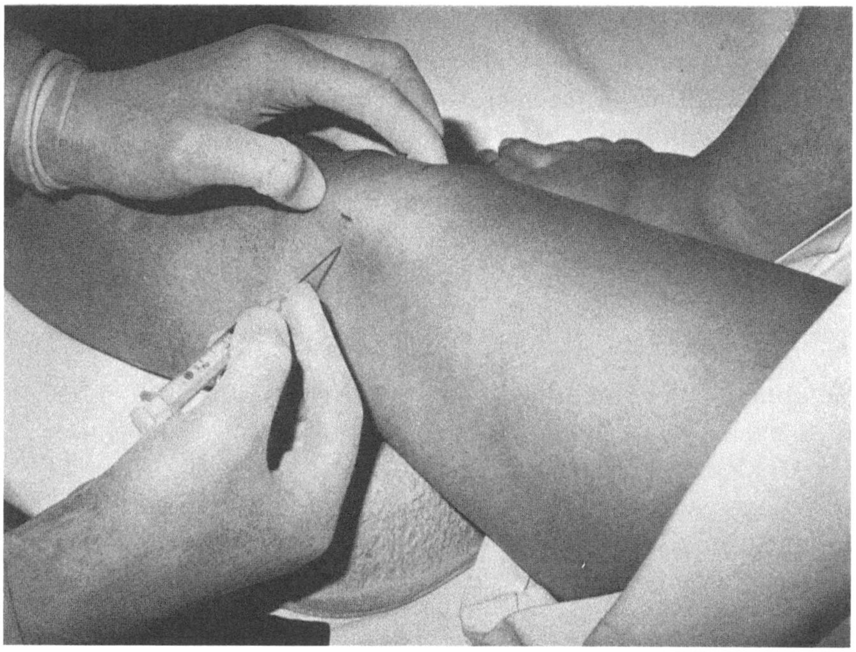

Fig. 3. Site of injection; the patella is moved laterally, the needle being introduced into the articular cavity at half the height of the patella and 1 cm dorsal to the lateral margin of the patella

2 ml syringe. A few milliliters of synovia can be removed with the small syringe, but a larger amount of synovia is more easily removed with a large syringe. Registration of the nature and amount of synovia removed is important. When no synovia is produced at puncture, the intra-articular position of the needle can be verified by injection of 2 ml air. Rapid injection of air usually causes some protrusion of soft tissue on the medial side. This procedure can be repeated when the first result is inconclusive. If soft tissue still fails to protrude on the medial side at this repetition, the entire puncture is best repeated. After verification of the intra-articular position of the needle, the positive contrast medium is injected. We use 5 ml 60% Urografin. The syringe used for the contrast medium is then filled with air and emptied into the joint. We use 30–40 ml air. Throughout the injection procedure, the left hand must keep the needle fixed in an absolutely unchanging position.

The needle is removed after injection of contrast medium and air, which are distributed through the intra-articular space by two slowly executed flexion-and-extension movements. Frequent, rapid flexion-and-extension movements promote foam formation within the joint (Fig. 66). It is unnecessary, and in fact inadvisable, to have the patient walk.

After the flexion-and-extension movements an elastic bandage is applied cranial to the patella so as to minimize accumulation of contrast media in the suprapatellar bursa. The puncture site is covered with a small piece of adhesive tape.

2.3 Arthrography

To obtain high-detail arthrograms, a fine-focus tube (0.15, 0.20, or 0.30 mm focus) should be used. A medium-high kilovoltage (70–90 kV) ensures adequate contrast of arthrograms. A serial cassette is indispensable for detail projections. It is advisable to inactivate temporarily the exposure automat, thus preventing marked variations in exposure. After gaining some experience, it is not difficult to determine exposure times for the various detail projections.

2.3.1 Cruciate Ligaments

The patient is seated on the table, with the knee in 90° flexion (cf. Chap. 5). In this lateral projection, the central beam extends horizontally and aims at the articular cavity of the knee. The patient, wearing leaded rubber gloves, holds the cassette (18 × 24 cm) beside the knee. The investigator, also wearing leaded rubber gloves, sits on the patient's foot and pulls the lower leg towards his own body. This ensures maximum extension of the anterior cruciate ligament (Figs. 4a and 127). The next exposure is made in a similar manner, but this time the investigator pushes against the lower leg, thus verifying intactness of the posterior cruciate ligament (Figs. 4b and 127). These two supplemental exposures usually provide adequate information on the cruciate ligament compartments.

2.3.2 Menisci

The examination starts with the medial meniscus, the patient lying on the side of the knee to be examined. At half the length of the lower leg, a shoulder support or other type of support has been attached to the table. The healthy leg lies on the ventral

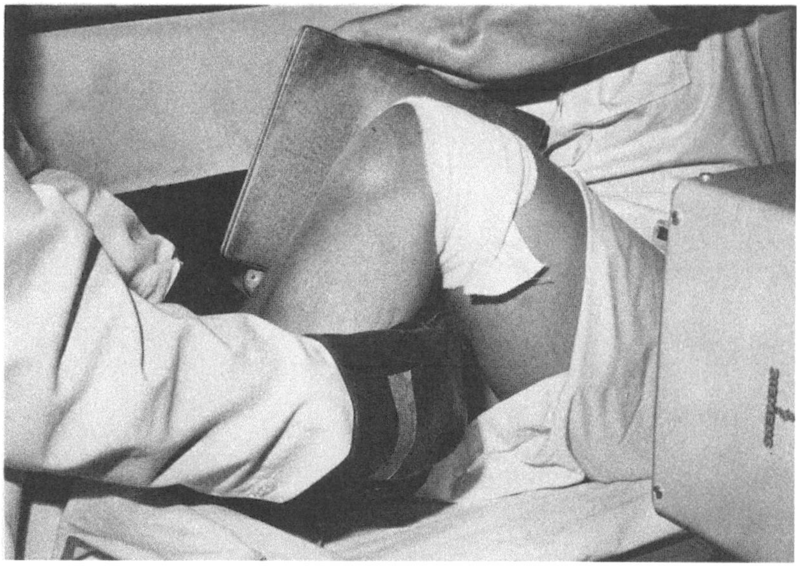

a

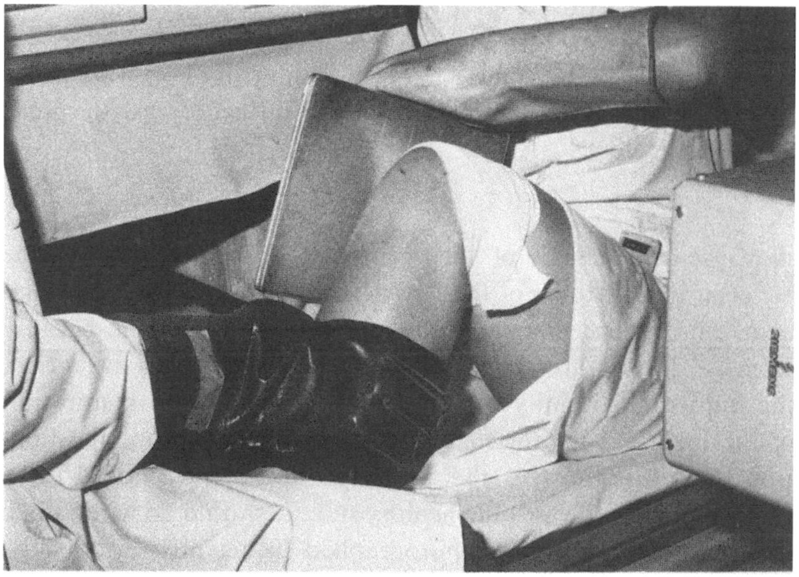

b

Fig. 4a and b. Arthrography of both cruciate ligaments with the knee in 90° flexion. (a) Arthrography of the anterior cruciate ligament, with traction applied to the lower leg. (b) Arthrography of the posterior cruciate ligament, with pressure applied to the lower leg

side of the leg to be examined (Fig. 5). The various detail projections of the medial anterior horn, midportion, and posterior horn are obtained by having the patient turn slightly more to the prone position after each exposure, while the investigator pushes the lower leg against the vertical support. Provided the patient keeps the knee entirely relaxed, the medial articular cavity is thus slightly dilatated. A careful eye should be kept on the

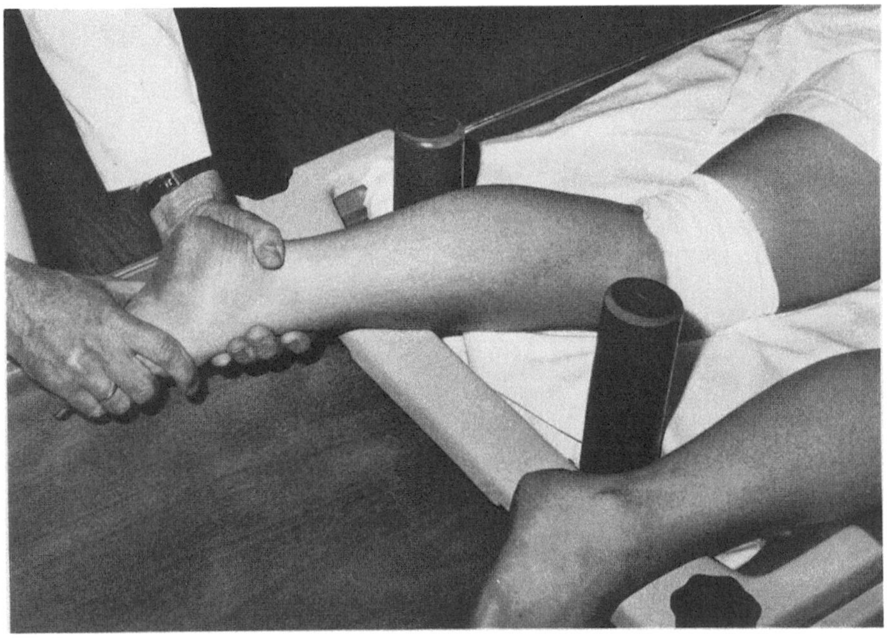

Fig. 5. Patient's position during examination of the medial meniscus. After each exposure the patient turns slightly further towards the prone position

sharp central margin of the meniscus, which becomes visible between the contours of the femoral condyle and the tibial plateau. The central margin of the meniscus is important, because meniscal lesions are not infrequently localized solely on, or in, the immediate vicinity of the central margin. The midportion of the meniscus is projected with the patient in prone position. For the projections of the posterior horn, the patient turns slightly further towards the healthy side. It should be ascertained that the posterior horn is photographed sufficiently far dorsally. A good landmark in this respect is the appearance of both condyles in this projection. In the majority of cases a series of 12 detail projections is sufficient for adequate examination of the entire medial meniscus (Figs. 18 and 19).

The lateral meniscus is examined with the patient prone and slightly on the healthy side. The vertical table support rests against the calf, halfway up the lower leg (Fig. 6). The lateral anterior horn, midportion, and posterior horn are in principle photographed in the same way as with the medial meniscus. Again the patient turns on his stomach and then slightly on the side to be examined. With the lateral meniscus, too, it must be ensured that the posterior horn is projected sufficiently far dorsally (Fig. 23).

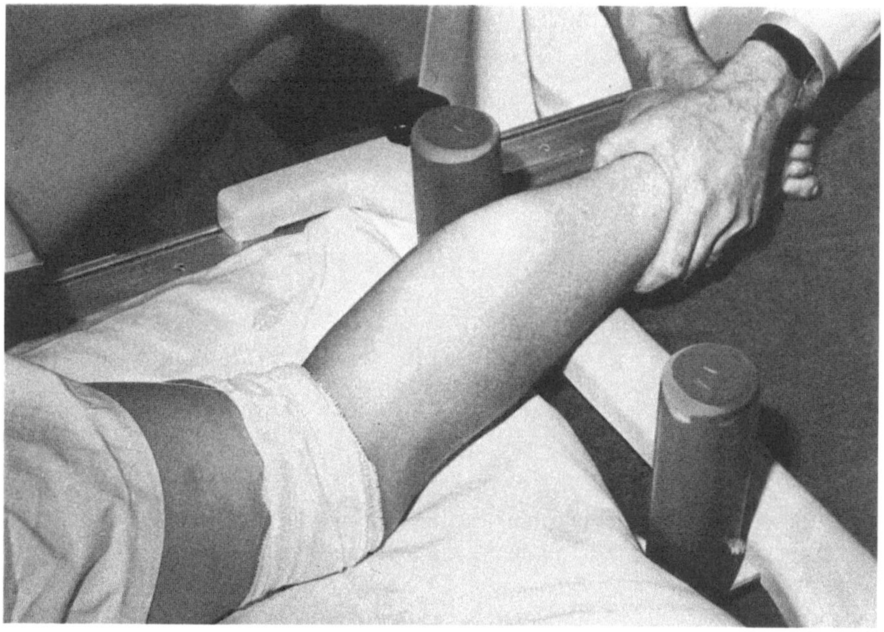

Fig. 6. Patient's position during examination of the lateral meniscus. After each exposure the patient turns slightly further towards the prone position

2.3.3 Patellofemoral Joint

Projections of the retropatellar area are of special importance in the diagnosis of retropatellar cartilaginous lesions.

2.3.3.1 Lateral Projections

In the lateral projections, evaluation of the medial and lateral aspects of the patella is difficult. With the knee joint slightly rotated, they project on the femoral condyles. The lateral examination is best done during active and/or passive hyperextension of the knee (Fig. 7). The cartilage of the patellar eminence is clearly depicted (Figs. 93 and 94).

2.3.3.2 Tangential Projections

With the patient seated, three tangential exposures are made while the patient successively flexes the knee 30°, 60°, and 90°. From the foot, the central beam extends at an angle of about 10° with the lower leg, and is aimed at the inferior aspect of the patella. The patient uses both hands to hold the lead-pro-

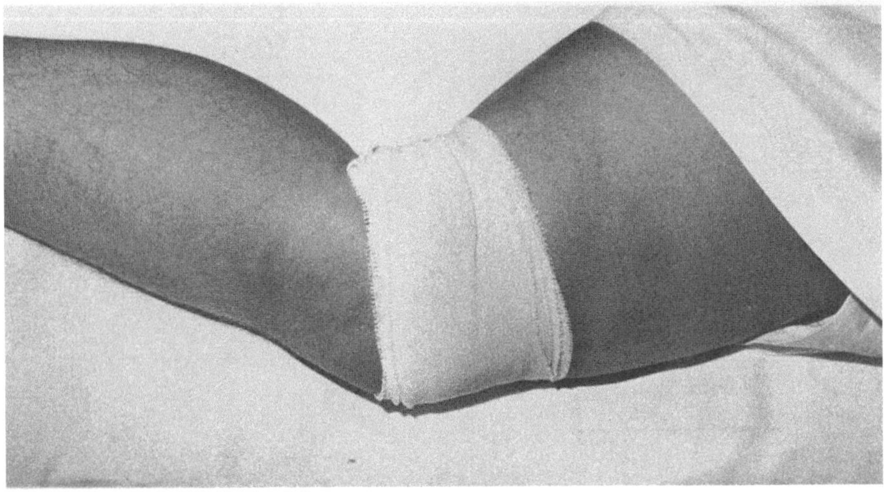

Fig. 7. Patient's position for lateral projections of the patellofemoral joint. The examination is best made during active and/or passive hyperextension of the knee

tected cassette in the correct position cranial to the knee joint (Fig. 8). Each of these three tangential exposures shows part of the medial and lateral aspects, thus giving a clear impression of the retropatellar cartilage surface (Fig. 92).
The experienced investigator can complete this arthrographic examination, including the injection procedure, in about 15–20 min. If carried out with technical accuracy, this double contrast arthrography is a valuable aid in the diagnosis of lesions of the cruciate ligaments and the menisci and degenerative cartilaginous lesions. The reliability of this method will later be discussed in detail.

2.4 Aftercare and Complications of Arthrography

After double contrast arthrography in the manner described, the bandage can be removed and the patient sent home. Because the synovium is bound to be irritated by the puncture and the injection of contrast medium and air, we advise the patient to be careful with the knee joint on the day of examination and the following day. Frequent flexion-and-extension movements (e.g., cycling) should be restricted. In a fair number of cases there are minor complaints about the knee joint examined: some hydrops and slight pain may persist for a few days but disappear spontaneously. Freiberger et al. (1966) performed synovial biop-

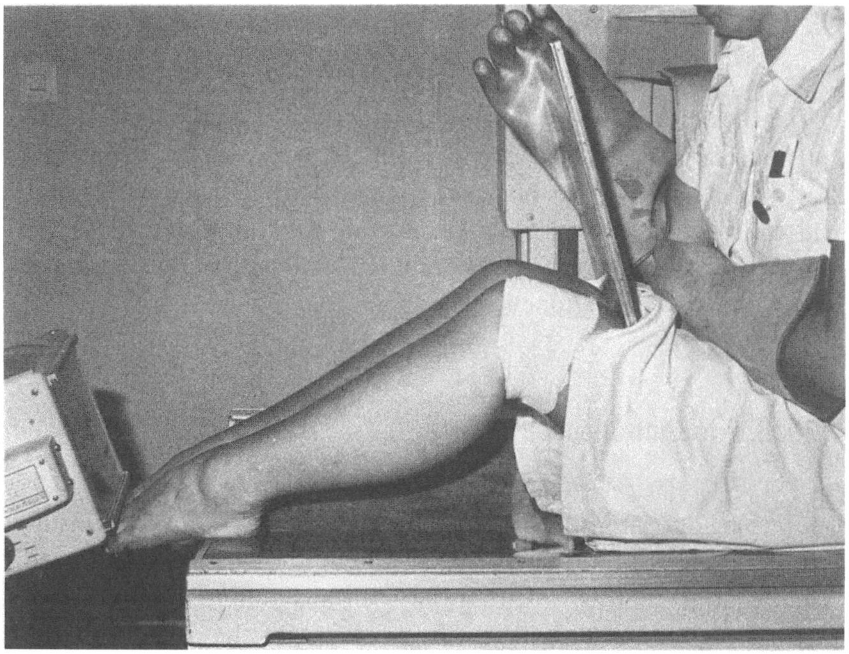

Fig. 8. Tangential projection of the patella. During routine double contrast arthrography these exposures are made at 30°, 60°, and 90° flexion of the knee. The central beam extends from the foot at an angle of about 10° with the lower leg and is aimed at the inferior margin of the patella

sies in 21 patients over a period of 1–3 months after double contrast arthrography. In none of these patients were histological changes resulting from the arthrography demonstrable.

Since after arthrography the radiologist loses sight of many patients, or sees them only after a considerable time, it is difficult to estimate the exact number of patients who develop complications after the examination.

2.4.1 Hydrops

Lindblom (1948) found hydrops of the knee joint in 5% of his patients; he had used 35% Perabrodil as contrast medium. Wiener (1967) reported hydrops in 3% of cases after using 50% Hypaque M or 60% Renografin. Hydrops results from abacterial synovitis. Roebuck (1977) compared 60% Urografin with Dimer X. With the latter, swelling of the knee joint and heat sensations were substantially less marked than with 60% Urografin. No other reports on this new contrast medium have so far been published.

2.4.2 Allergic Reactions

Nicholas et al. (1970) reported four urticarial reactions in 3,000 arthrograms using 60% Renografin. In our own case material of 4,000 patients, we observed one urticarial reaction, 15 min after injection of 5 ml 60% Urografin. Ricklin et al. (1971) reported one case of urticaria combined with asthmatic symptoms and one case of angioneurotic edema.

2.4.3 Air Embolism

Double contrast arthrography, in which the amount of air insufflated is substantially smaller than the amount of gas introduced in negative contrast arthrography, entails only a minimal risk of air embolism. Of course, after rupture of the capsule or the ligaments, air can readily enter the muscles. Wiener (1967) described a patient who, probably as a result of this, developed pneumo-mediastinum.

2.4.4 Arthritis

This is a very serious complication, caused by inadequate aseptic and antiseptic measures prior to puncture of the joint. This complication of course calls for intensive antibiotic medication.

The low incidence of serious complications after double contrast arthrography justifies an ample range of indication. Carefully performed double contrast arthrography gives exact information on intra-articular structures. Test arthrotomy is obsolete. Repetition of arthrographic examination in cases of doubt is certainly justifiable.

3 Meniscal Lesions

3.1 Specific Anatomy

The menisci are localized between the cartilage surfaces of the two femoral condyles and the tibial plateau (Fig. 9). They are crescent shaped and consist mainly of fibrocartilaginous tissue and elastic fibers, most of which are arranged longitudinally. The menisci are connected to the capsule, the zone of transition between menisci and capsule consisting of low-density connective tissue. Extensions of the capsule form the coronary ligaments which connect the meniscal margins to the underlying tibial surface. From the capsule, small blood vessels enter the outer one-third of the menisci, especially in the midportion. The peripheral one-third of the anterior and the posterior horn is least vascularized. The vascularization of the lateral meniscus is slightly more extensive than that of the medial meniscus.

3.1.1 Medial Meniscus

The curvature of the medial meniscus is less marked than that of the lateral meniscus. The former follows the margins of the tibial plateau and is wedge shaped in cross section. Gaillard (1966) studied the width and height of the menisci in adult subjects and found that the *width* of the medial anterior horn is 8–10 mm and that of the posterior horn is 16–20 mm. Eikelaar (1975) found that the *thickness* of the medial meniscus at the site of the capsule insertion is 16–17 mm in the area of the posterior horn and 8–9 mm in that of the anterior horn. Gaillard found a thickness of 5–7 mm in his anatomic specimens.
The fixation of the medial anterior horn is fourfold. Fibers of the medial anterior horn connect with the anterior margin of the tibia and with the ventral margin of the intercondylar eminence. In addition there is usually a fibrous connection with the anterior cruciate ligament, and the transverse ligament con-

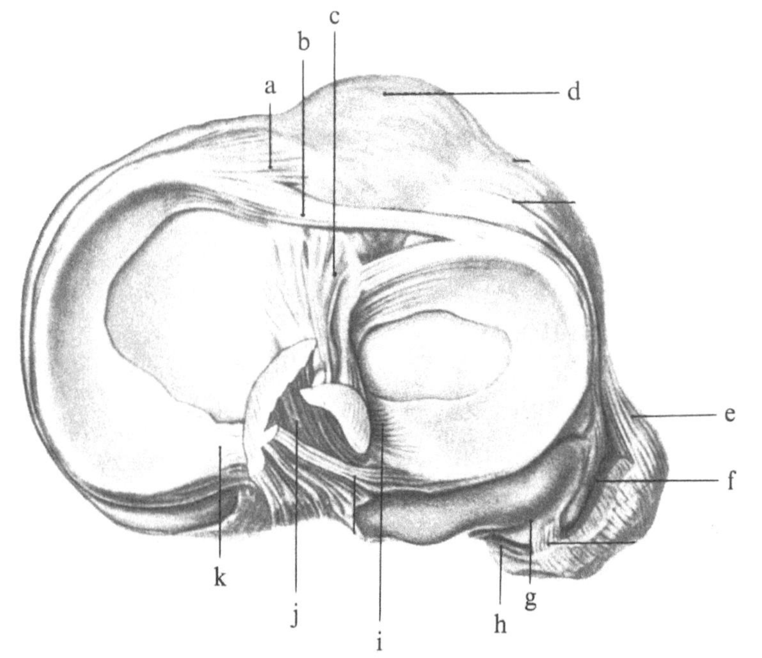

a. Crus anterius menisci medialis
b. Ligamentum transversum genu
c. Ligamentum cruciatum anterius
d. Tuberositas tibiae
e. Ligamentum capitis fibulae anterius
f. Articulatio tibiofibularis
g. Sulcus m. poplitei
h. Recessus subpopliteus
i. Crus posterius menisci lateralis
j. Lig. cruciatum posterius
k. Crus posterius menisci medialis

Fig. 9a. Tibial plateau, menisci and cruciate ligaments (Lanz and Wachsmuth, 1972)

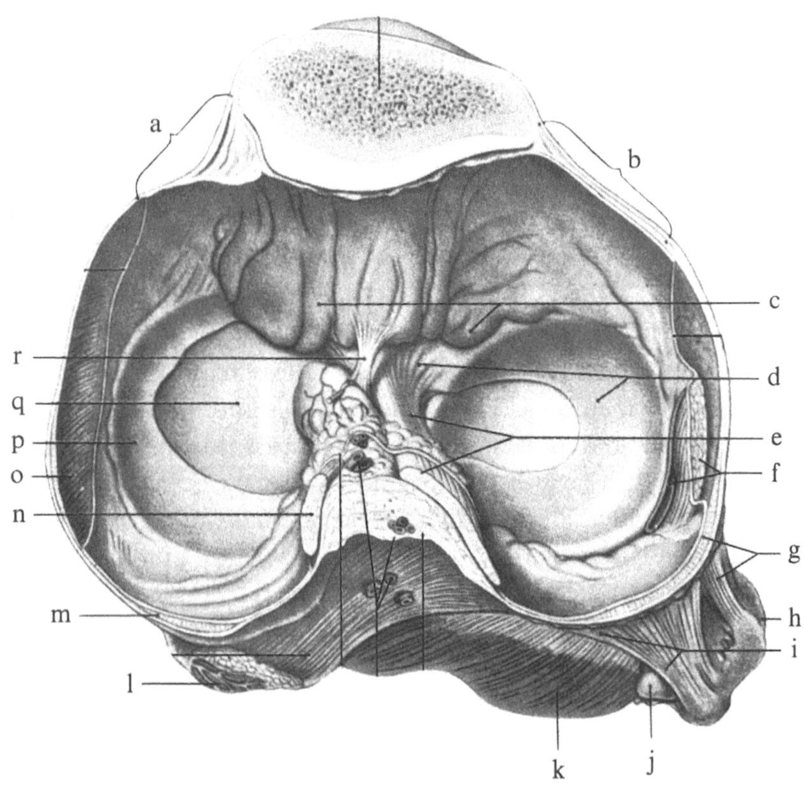

a. Retinaculum patellae mediale
b. Retinaculum patellae laterale
c. Plicae alares
d. Crus anterius menisci lateralis et meniscus lateralis
e. Ligamentum cruciatum anterius
f. Tendo musculus poplitei
g. Ligamentum collaterale laterale
h. Caput fibulae
i. Ligamentum popliteum arcuatum et retinaculum
j. Bursa musculi poplitei
k. Musculus popliteus
l. Musculus semimembranosus
m. Caput mediale musculus gastrocnemii
n. Ligamentum cruciatum posterius
o. Ligamentum collaterale mediale
p. Meniscus medialis
q. Condylus medialis tibiae
r. Plica synovialis infrapatellaris

Fig. 9b. Articular cavity of the knee and soft tissues. The patella is in cross section (Lanz and Wachsmuth, 1972) nects the medial anterior horn to the lateral anterior horn. At the sites of contact between meniscus and capsule, there is a firm connection with the capsule and therefore with the medial collateral ligament. The posterior horn of the medial meniscus connects to the bony area immediately behind the intercondylar eminence. This site of insertion lies between the sites of insertion of the posterior horn of the lateral meniscus and the posterior cruciate ligament.

3.1.2 Lateral Meniscus

This has a smaller radius of curvature and consequently is nearly annular. In cross section, the lateral meniscus is likewise wedge shaped, having a concave upper surface and a slightly convex undersurface. Measurements made by Gaillard (1966) indicate a width of 12–13 mm (variation 2–3 mm). The thickness of the lateral meniscus is 7–8 mm in the midportion, while the anterior and the posterior horn are 2–3 mm less thick. Eikelaar (1975) reported a thickness of 11–13 mm.

The lateral anterior horn inserts near the intercondylar eminence. As already mentioned, there is a connection with the medial anterior horn via the transverse ligament. The lateral posterior horn connects to the bone behind the intercondylar eminence immediately anterior to the site of insertion of the medial posterior horn. A few fibers of the posterior horn continue into the posterior cruciate ligament as meniscifibular ligament. The connection of the lateral meniscus with the capsule is less firm.

On the ventrolateral side there is a tissue bridge between meniscus and capsule. In the posterior horn the bridge between meniscus and capsule is interrupted by the tendon sheath of the popliteal muscle. The latter arises from the posterior aspect of the tibia. The insertion of the tendon is a complex structure. The superficial part of the popliteal muscle connects to the lateral margin of the lateral posterior horn. In a few cases the superficial fibers continue into the tendon of the popliteal muscle. That is why this part of the meniscus is not usually in contact with the lateral femoral condyle. Deeper fibers of the popliteal muscle continue into the joint capsule near the lateral femoral condyle and insert immediately below the collateral ligament. According to Last (1948, 1950), the popliteal muscle is enclosed in a sheath of which the lateral wall is formed by the fibrous capsule, while the medial wall is formed by the synovial membrane. Consequently the tendon of the popliteal muscle could not be free in the intra-articular space. Eikelaar (1975) reported that the tendon of the popliteal muscle is clearly visible in the intra-articular space by arthroscopy.

3.2. Meniscal Functions

The literature ascribes the following functions to the menisci:
1) The menisci jointly form a cushion or buffer between femur and tibia, causing the pressure of the femur to be distributed over a larger tibial surface and thus enhancing the elasticity of the joint. Together with the ligaments of the joint, they form a single functional unit. The pressure experiments which Maquet (1976) carried out with cadaver knees clearly confirmed this theory. In a test arrangement with an isolated knee joint in 90° flexion and with 225 kg pressure on the distal part of the femur, the weight-bearing tibial plateau surface measured 11.5 cm^2. Removal of the menisci reduced this surface to 5.6 cm^2.
These experiments demonstrate the efficacy of the menisci. Removal of a meniscus causes greatly increased pressure per square centimeter of tibial plateau, and this of course facilitates development of arthrotic changes. Fairbank (1948), for example, presented radiographs showing various lesions that had mainly occurred after meniscectomy; he ascribed these lesions to abolition of the weight-bearing function of the menisci. An in vitro study made by Walker and Hajek (1972) showed that the menisci enlarge the weight-bearing area, particularly in the extreme mobility areas of the knee. On the basis of a study of human and porcine knees, Shrive (1974) calculated that the menisci account for 40%–60% of weight-bearing.
2) The menisci distribute the synovial fluid required for nutrition of the articulating surfaces of femur and tibia.
3) The menisci facilitate adequate lubrication of the femorotibial joint (MacConaill, 1932; King, 1936).
4) The menisci prevent incarceration of capsule and synovial membrane during knee movements (Eikelaar, 1975).
5) The menisci are of functional importance for optimal rotation on a vertical axis within the knee joint (Kaplan, 1955).
6) The menisci enhance the stability of the knee in that they deepen the articulating joint surfaces and fill the dead space between femoral condyles and tibial plateau (Brantigan and Voshell 1941, 1943; Walker and Erkman, 1975; Eikelaar, 1975).

The above mentioned meniscal functions show clearly that unnecessary excision of one or both menisci is to be avoided.

3.3 Friction and Lubrication

The joints are able to function quite well for years, in spite of the high intra-articular pressures which can occur with excessive use. This is possible only if friction and lubrication are well balanced. The coefficient of friction is a constant which indicates the relation between the force required to cause relative displacement of two objects and the force with which these objects are pressed together. The magnitude of this constant is dependent on the materials used, and especially on lubrication. Five different mechanisms of lubrication can be distinguished (Rijnks, 1976).

3.3.1 Interface Lubrication

The two articular surfaces are in contact; friction is reduced by the presence of a thin layer of molecules on the articular surface.

3.3.2 Buffer Lubrication

A layer of fluid is temporarily present between the articular surfaces and is pressed away when stress is applied. The film of fluid can temporarily absorb force because in the articular cavity there is resistance to escape of the fluid.

3.3.3 Elastohydrodynamic Lubrication

The articular surfaces are separated by a film of fluid. This film is determined by the shape and the relative velocities of the articular surfaces in relation to the film.

3.3.4 Sponge Lubrication

Under functional stress, fluid, which lubricates, is pressed out of the cartilage.

3.3.5 Lubrication by a Transient Increase in Viscosity

The synovia lubricates. It can be regarded as a dialysate of blood plasma with hyaluronic acid, a polysaccharide with a molecular weight of about 3,800,000. Interface lubrication could result from adhesion of the hyaluronic acid to the cartilaginous surface. The protein fraction is believed to play an important role in this respect (Maroudas, 1968a, b; MacCutchen, 1966; Linn, 1968).
The problem of lubrication in synovial joints has prompted much experimental research. Rijnks (1976) concluded that, in view of the data available in the literature, a combination of several mechanisms of lubrication is plausible.
Although in degenerative arthropathies changes have been found in the chemical and mechanical properties of the synovia, their influence on the lubricant properties remains obscure.

3.4 Etiology of Meniscal Lesions

3.4.1 Mobility of the Menisci

The menisci move dorsally at flexion and ventrally at extension of the knee joint. The meniscal displacement is passively caused by the movements of the femoral condyle. At exorotation of the tibia, the posterior horn of the medial meniscus remains in the posterior part of the joint. The anterior horn is extended and pulled centrally, while the lateral meniscus slides forward. At endorotation of the tibia the medial meniscus slides forward in relation to the tibia, while the posterior horn is extended. The lateral meniscus remains behind, and its anterior horn is extended (Kingma, 1955). Since during rotations in the knee joint the menisci move together with the condyle over the tibial plateau, abnormal forces are produced, particularly between the undersurface of the menisci and the tibial plateau, thus often causing ruptures of the menisci in the undersurface (Smillie, 1975).

Smillie (1974) maintained that the lateral meniscus is more mobile than the medial meniscus because the fixation points of the posterior and the anterior horn are much closer together, giving the meniscus a marked radius of curvature. Secondly, the lateral meniscus can actively be moved dorsally by the popliteal muscle, because superficial fibers of this muscle are connected to the posterior horn. Moreover, the lateral meniscus is locally connected to the capsule but not to the collateral ligament.
The medial meniscus shows a higher incidence of ruptures than the lateral meniscus. MacMurray (1948) and Heinold (1965) explained this by the close relations between medial meniscus and medial collateral ligament. According to Last (1950), the medial meniscus is twisted during femoral rotatory movements because the anterior and the posterior horn are fused with the tibia and the midportion moves along via the collateral ligament. When the knee is flexed with the lower leg in fixed position, endorotation of the femur pulls the medial meniscus back. This displacement of the medial meniscus is counteracted by the elasticity of the medial meniscus, the firm fixation to capsule and collateral ligament, and the insertion of the posterior and the anterior horn on the tibial plateau.
Due to the much less marked fixation of the lateral meniscus to the capsule, its mobility is greater, and this is probably why ruptures of the lateral meniscus are less frequently observed. However, transverse ruptures of the lateral meniscus are more frequent. According to Ricklin et al. (1964, 1971), transverse ruptures result from marked displacement and hyperextension of the meniscus. Transverse rupture is believed to occur more readily due to the marked radius of curvature of the lateral meniscus.
To summarize: Particularly a combination of vigorous flexion-and-extension movements and rotatory movements is an important mechanical factor in the etiology of meniscal lesions. The normal mobility of the menisci is affected, and abnormal tensile and compressive forces develop which exceed the limit of elasticity of the menisci.

3.4.2 Risk-Increasing Factors

Congenital meniscal lesions mostly involve the lateral meniscus and often take the form of a discoid meniscus. Incarceration of a discoid meniscus can lead to degenerative lesions and ruptures (cf. p. 43).

A flaccid musculature and flaccid ligaments of the knee joint cause less firm fixation of the menisci, which are therefore more vulnerable to injury. Fresh or old ruptures of the collateral ligaments and/or cruciate ligaments, for example, cause increased mobility within the joint, and this can provoke meniscal lesions. Meniscal ganglions (cystic degeneration) are observed mainly in the lateral meniscus. Incisures are often visible, and not infrequently the process also involves the capsule. The mobility of the lateral meniscus is reduced, and the risk of rupture increases. Fatty degeneration of the cartilage cells leads to reduced elasticity and increases the risk of rupture. Macroscopically, these menisci show a spotted, yellowish surface with small fissures and ruptures (cf. 4.3.1).

Occupations which involve much squatting or kneeling increase the risk of meniscal lesions. Inhabitants of mountainous areas and miners are often exposed to microtraumata, which may explain the high rate of meniscal degeneration observed in these groups. These degenerations increase the risk of rupture. In miners, it is believed, prolonged squatting causes the synovia to be pressed away between condyles and menisci. At extension of the knee, the posterior horn of the medial meniscus becomes incarcerated between the condyles and can rupture (Kingma, 1955). Such sports as football and skiing are also notorious for a high incidence of meniscal ruptures.

3.5 Normal Radiologic Anatomy of the Menisci

3.5.1 Medial Meniscus

The meniscus is crescent shaped. Detail projections show a triangular cross section, the upper surface and undersurface being covered by a thin layer of positive contrast medium which contrasts sharply with the adjacent air. At the site of fixation of the medial meniscus to the capsule, contrast medium is of course not normally visible. The upper surface of the meniscus is slightly concave, corresponding to the convexity of the femoral condyle. The undersurface of the meniscus is slightly convex, corresponding to the concavity of the tibial plateau. Interindividual differences in width and height of the meniscus are known. A recess is often observed at the transition from medial meniscus to capsule, both on the superior and on the inferior aspect (Figs. 10

Fig. 10. Recess of the articular cavity between the superior aspect of the meniscus and the capsule

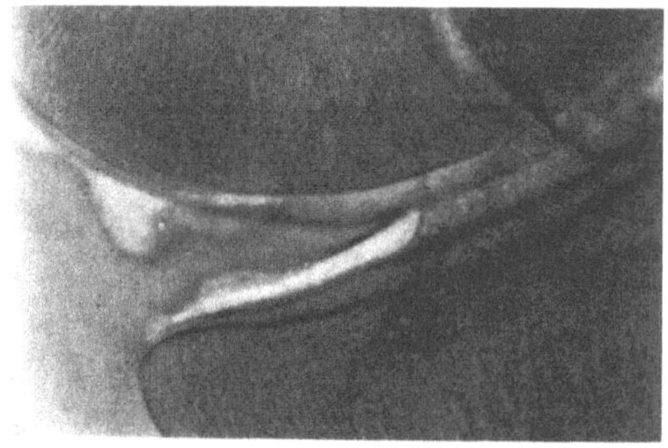

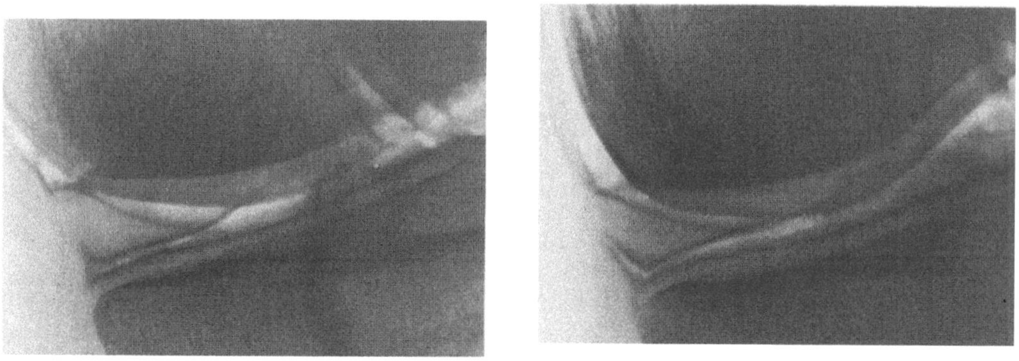

Fig. 11. Medial meniscus. Discontinuity between meniscus and capsule. Recess? Rupture? No arthroscopic lesion

and 22). According to Hall (1976), partial incisure of the posterior horn on the inferior aspect can produce features reminiscent of a recess (Fig. 11). If such an incisure is localized in the vascularized part of the meniscus, partial recovery is possible, which leaves a small, sharply defined recess. Detail projections of the medial anterior horn show the infrapatellar synovial fold (mucous ligament), which connects the Hoffa body to the intercondylar fossa (Figs. 12 and 132). Differentiation from a locally hypertrophic synovium or a flocculus of adipose tissue of the Hoffa body poses no difficulty (Figs. 13 and 150). Another possibility is that the entire Hoffa body is markedly swollen so that the medial anterior horn in the most ventral parts does not fully appear (Figs. 14 and 149). The hypertrophic flocculi of the Hoffa body and synovium and the infrapatellar synovial fold should not be mistaken for a ruptured and reversed part of the meniscus (Fig. 15). Virtually transverse projections of the anterior horn area can depict both the medial and the lateral anterior horn. Since the lateral anterior horn inserts more dorsally, the lateral horn in such cases is depicted behind the medial anterior horn (Fig. 16).

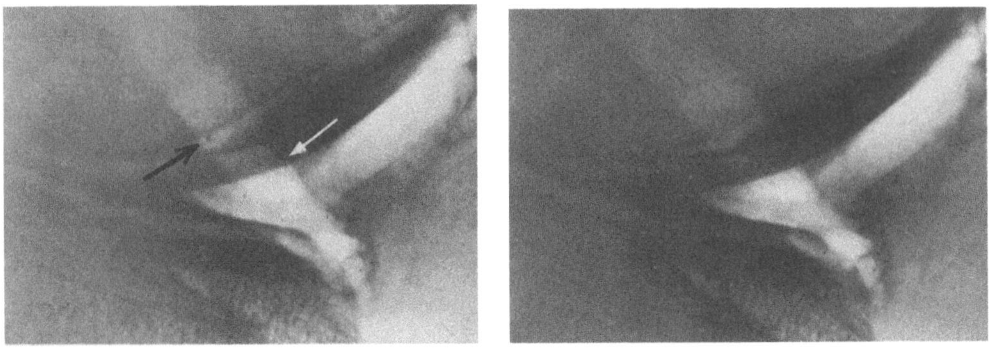

Fig. 12. Details of the medial anterior aspect of the joint. Delimitation of the anterior cruciate ligament (*black arrow*) and of the infrapatellar synovial fold (*white arrow*)

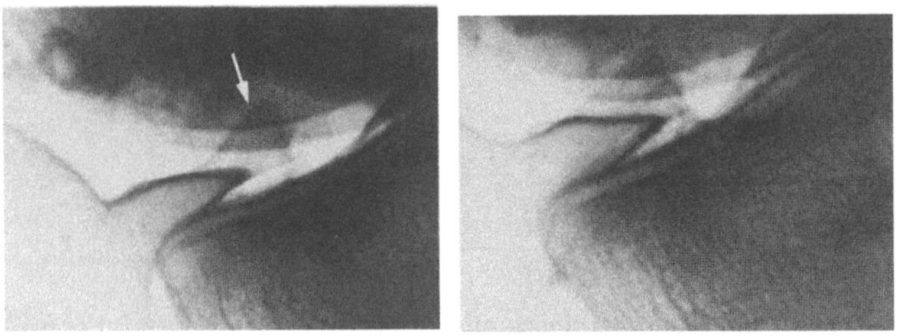

Fig. 13. Details of the anterior horn of the medial meniscus. Hypertrophic flake of synovial tissue (*arrow*)

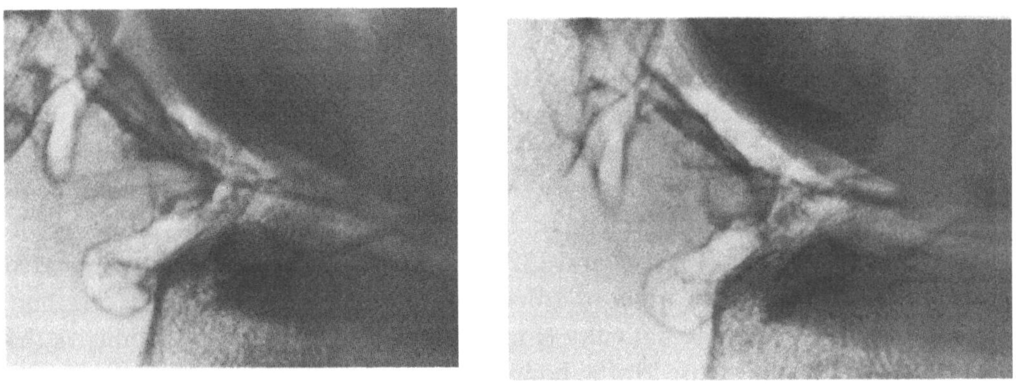

Fig. 14. Swollen Hoffa body partly concealing the central parts of the medial meniscus

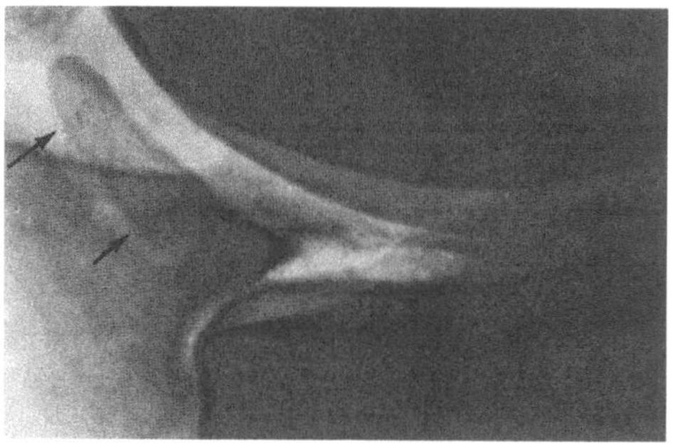

Fig. 15. Lesion of the medial meniscus with reverted part of the meniscus projected obliquely above the meniscus (*arrows*)

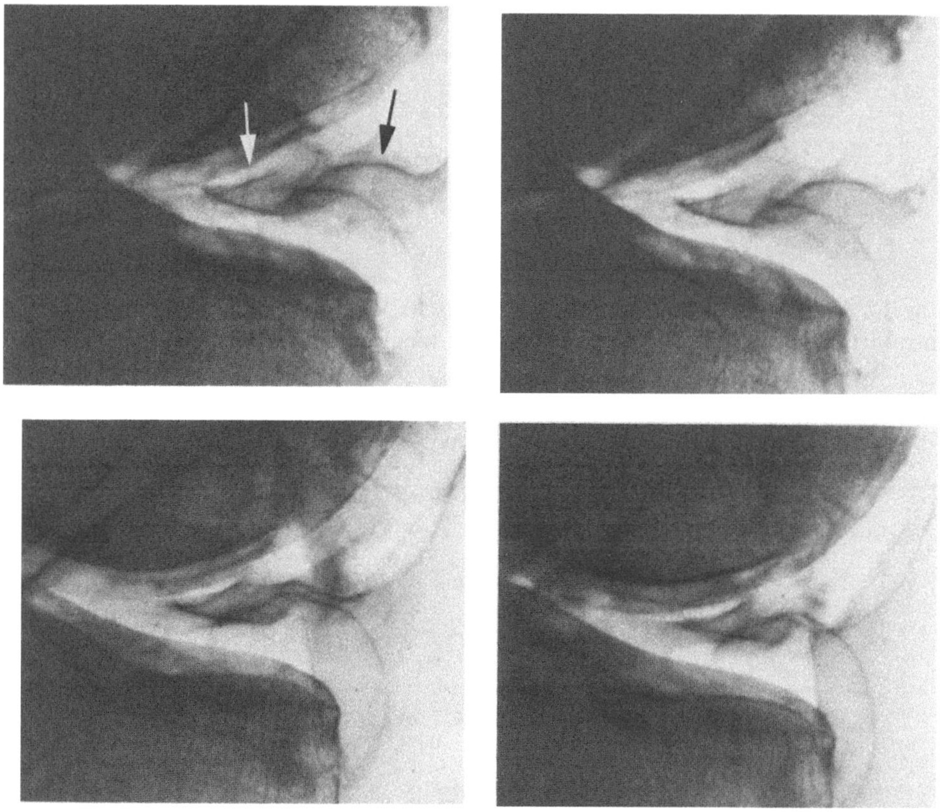

Fig. 16. Exposures of the lateral anterior aspect of the knee joint. Simultaneous projection of the lateral anterior horn (*white arrow*) and the medial anterior horn (*black arrow*)

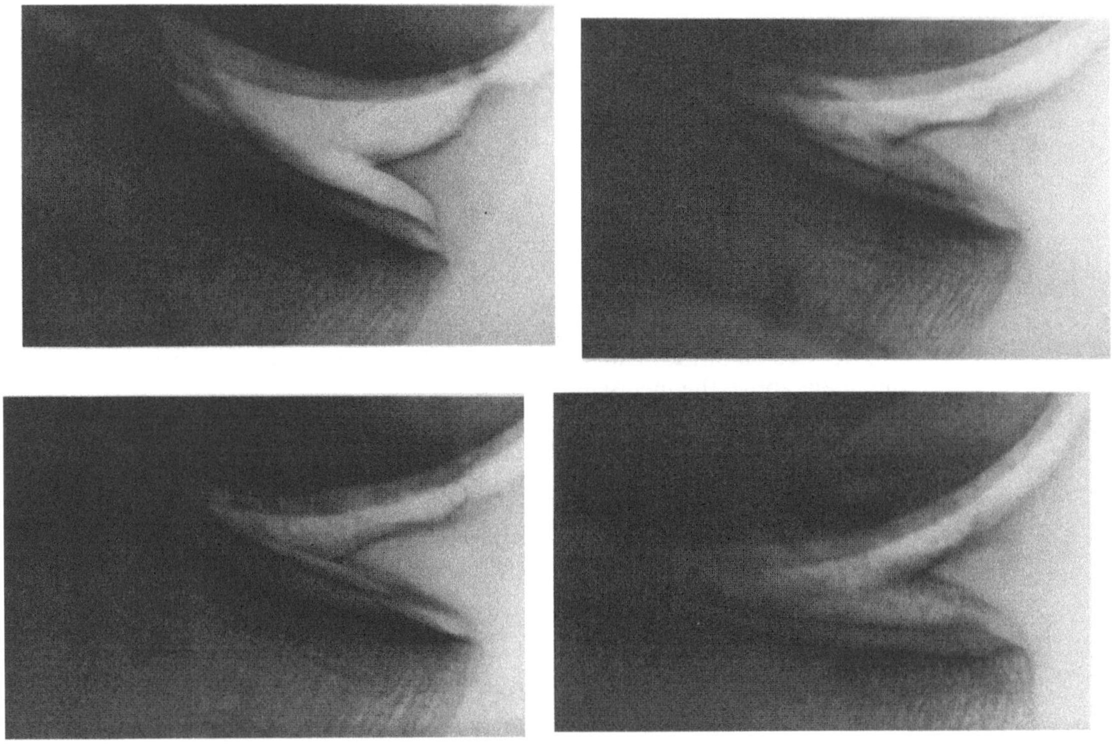

Fig. 17. Exposures of the same medial meniscus. Flaccid medial collateral ligament. The medial intra-articular space is dilatated. The medial meniscus is intact

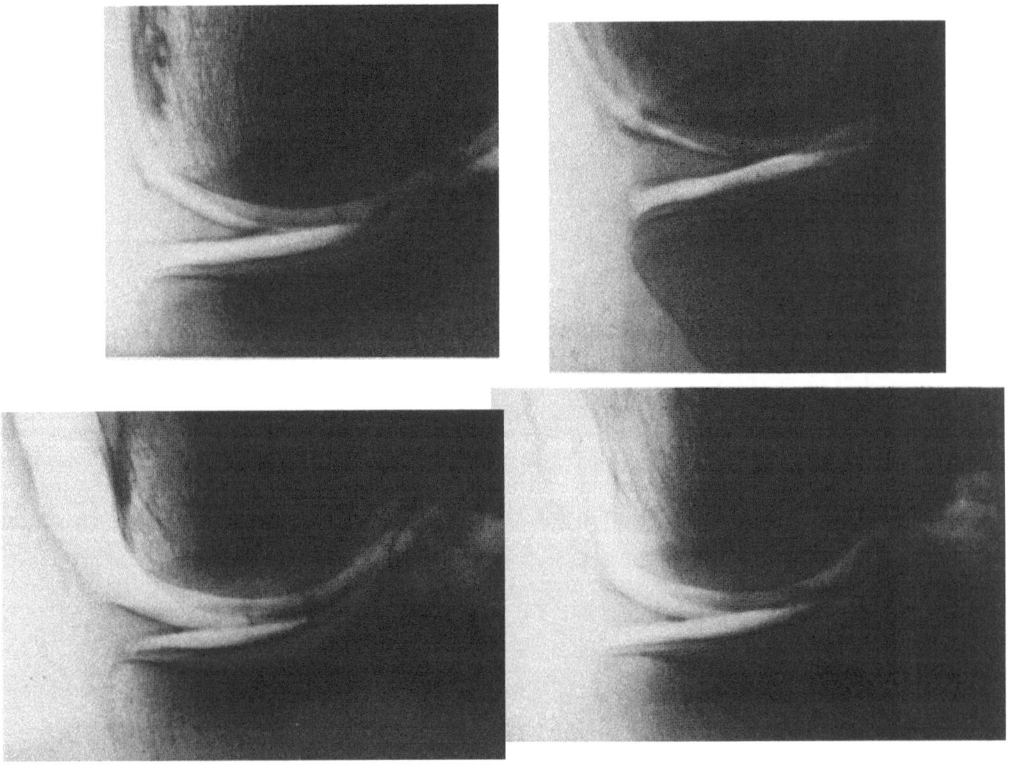

Fig. 18. Projections of the normal midportion of medial meniscus. The sharp central meniscus margin is projected quite free between femoral condyle and tibial plateau

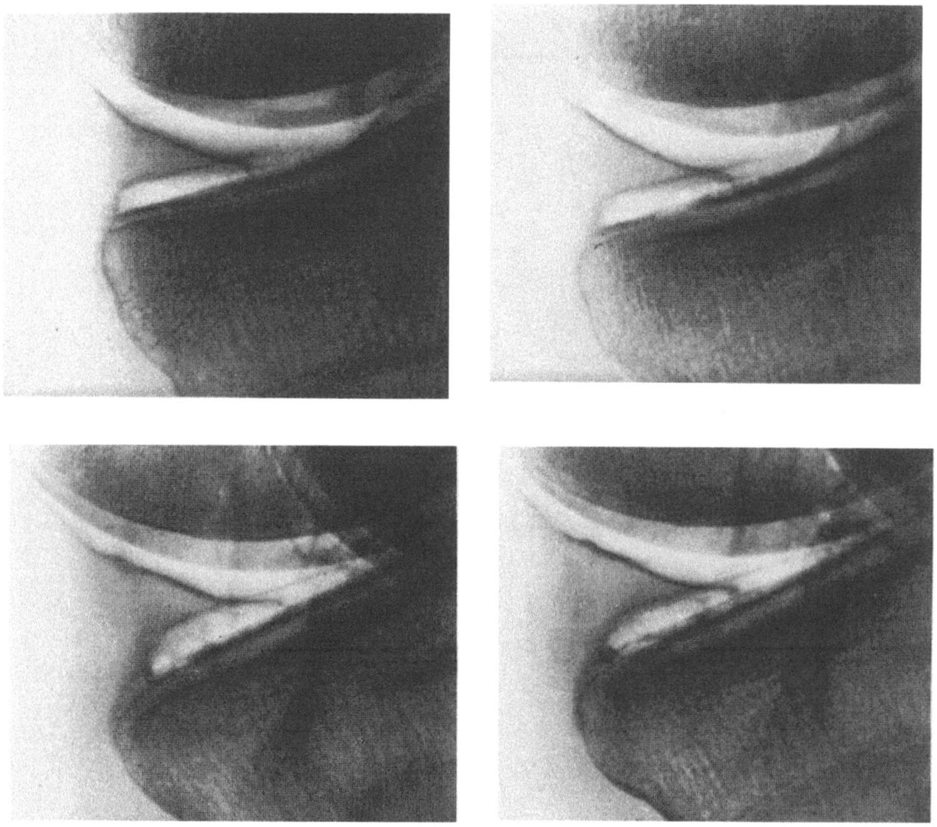

Fig. 19. Projections of the normal posterior horn of the medial meniscus. Sharply defined contours of femoral condyle, tibial plateau, and meniscus

When the medial collateral ligament is flaccid, the medial articular cavity is often extra wide, even though the meniscus can be entirely intact (Fig. 17). With an adequate arthrographic technique, giving attention to sufficient dilatation of the medial articular cavity and good projection of the central meniscal margin between femoral condyle and tibial plateau, the central margin of the meniscus should be sharply defined (Figs. 18 and 19). An irregular central margin is abnormal. This will be discussed in detail later. In the region of the medial posterior horn, a depiction of the semimembranosogastrocnemial bursa is regularly visible (cf. p. 128). The entry to the bursa is often also arthrographically visible (Figs. 20–22).

3.5.2 Normal Lateral Meniscus

The more annular lateral meniscus is of course also wedge shaped in cross section. It is broader than the medial meniscus, and less thick. Lateral projections of the anterior horn region can

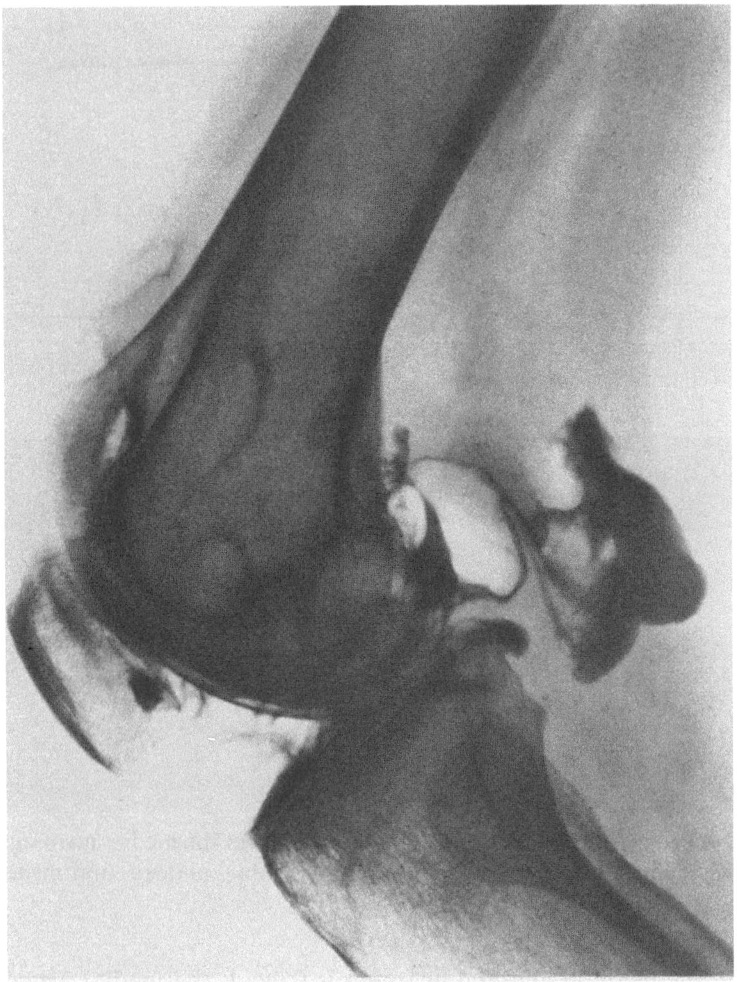

Fig. 20. Semimembranosogastrocnemial bursa. The communication with the articular cavity is clearly visible

depict both the medial and the lateral anterior horn (Fig. 16). The transition from meniscus to capsule is smooth (Fig. 23). The depicted lateral posterior horn differs essentially from the depicted medial posterior horn due to differences in anatomy. The tendon sheath of the popliteal muscle passes obliquely between the lateral posterior horn and the capsule so that arthrograms show only a narrow bridge of tissue between lateral posterior horn and capsule (Figs. 24 and 25). Other detail projections show no sign of any distinct connection at this level (Fig. 26). The tendon of the popliteal muscle is visible in the tendon sheath on several arthrograms. In two of the patients we examined, no tendon sheath proved demonstrable in the region of the lateral posterior horn. We have so far been unable to explain this.

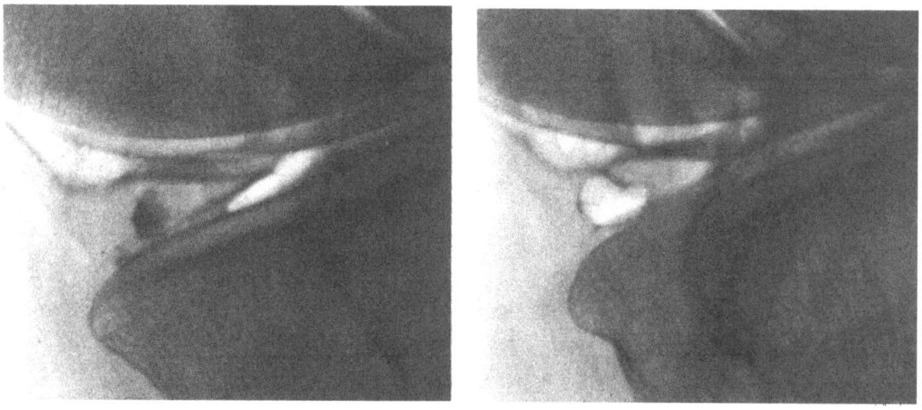

a b

Fig. 21a and b. Communication between the semimembranosogastrocnemial bursa and the articular cavity. (a) The communication is visualized by positive contrast medium. (b) The communication in double contrast

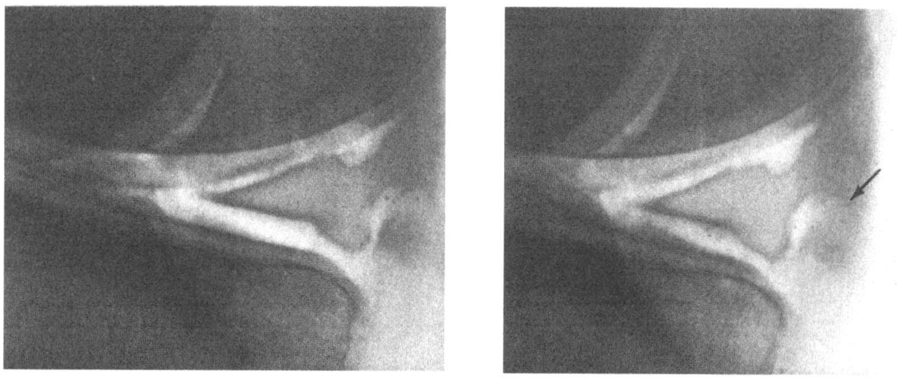

Fig. 22. Normal medial posterior horn. Recess of the articular cavity on the superior side of the meniscus. On the inferior side, the comunication between semimembranosogastrocnemial bursa and articular cavity is visible (*arrow*)

In the further course of the lateral meniscus the tendon sheath was also unobserved. In these patients, a solid connection proved to exist between lateral posterior horn and capsule (Figs. 27 and 28). In some cases the inferior capsular space communicates with the articular cavity of the tibiofibular joint via the popliteal tendon sheath and popliteal bursa (Figs. 29 and 166).

3.5.3 Spurious Meniscal Lesions

A not entirely freely projected central meniscal margin can impress as a rupture of the central part of the meniscus – a spurious

a

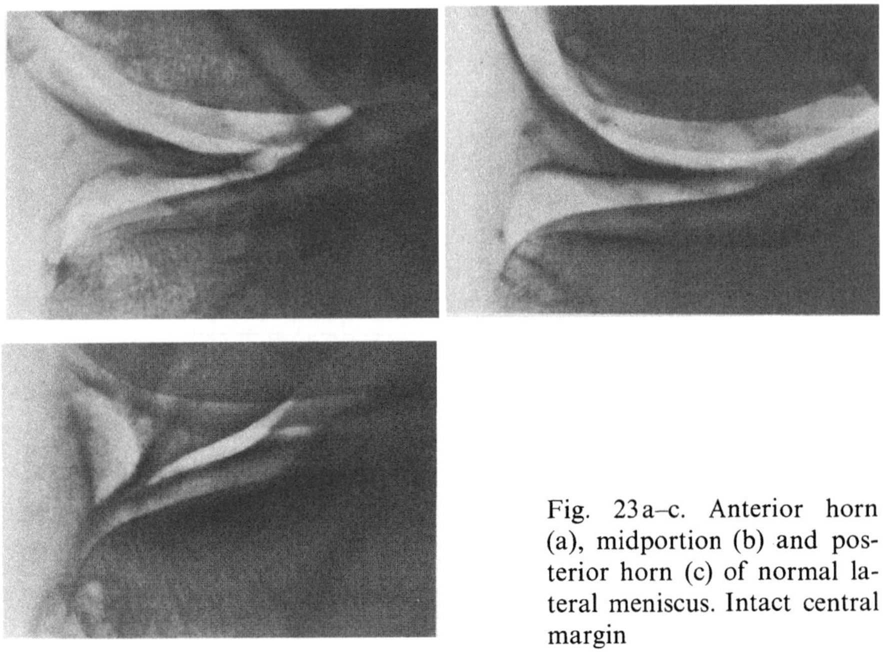

b

c

Fig. 23a–c. Anterior horn (a), midportion (b) and posterior horn (c) of normal lateral meniscus. Intact central margin

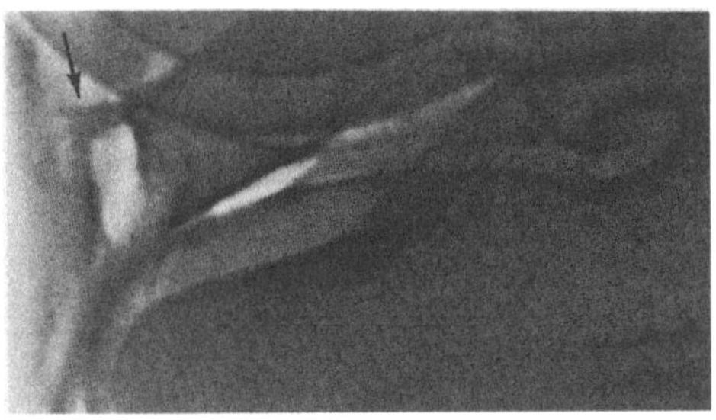

Fig. 24. Normal lateral posterior horn. Narrow bridge of tissue between meniscus and capsule at the top (*arrow*)

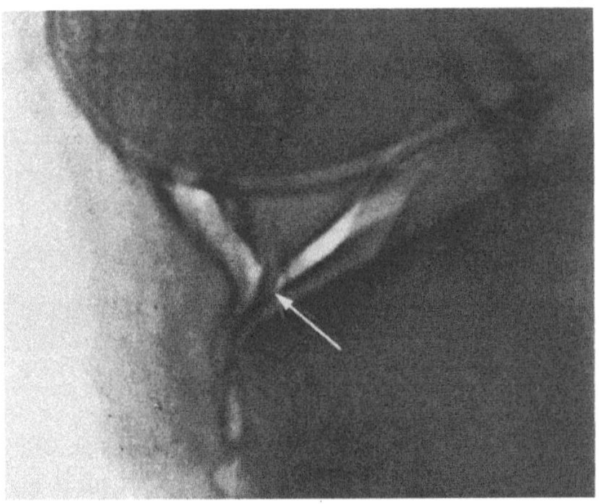

Fig. 25. Normal lateral posterior horn. Narrow bridge of tissue between meniscus and capsule at the bottom (*arrow*)

Fig. 26. Normal lateral posterior horn. Hardly any visible tissue bridge between lateral posterior horn and capsule

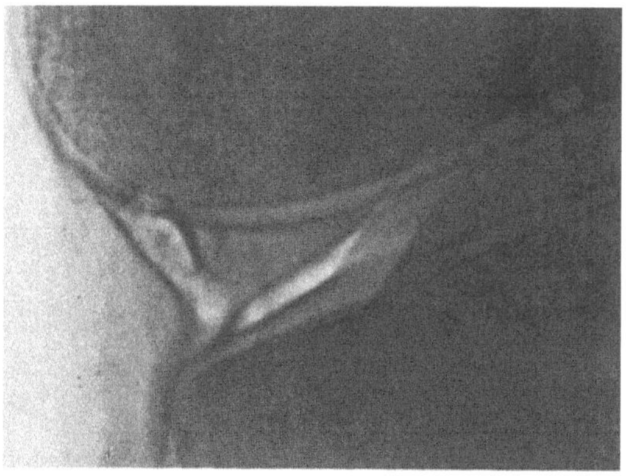

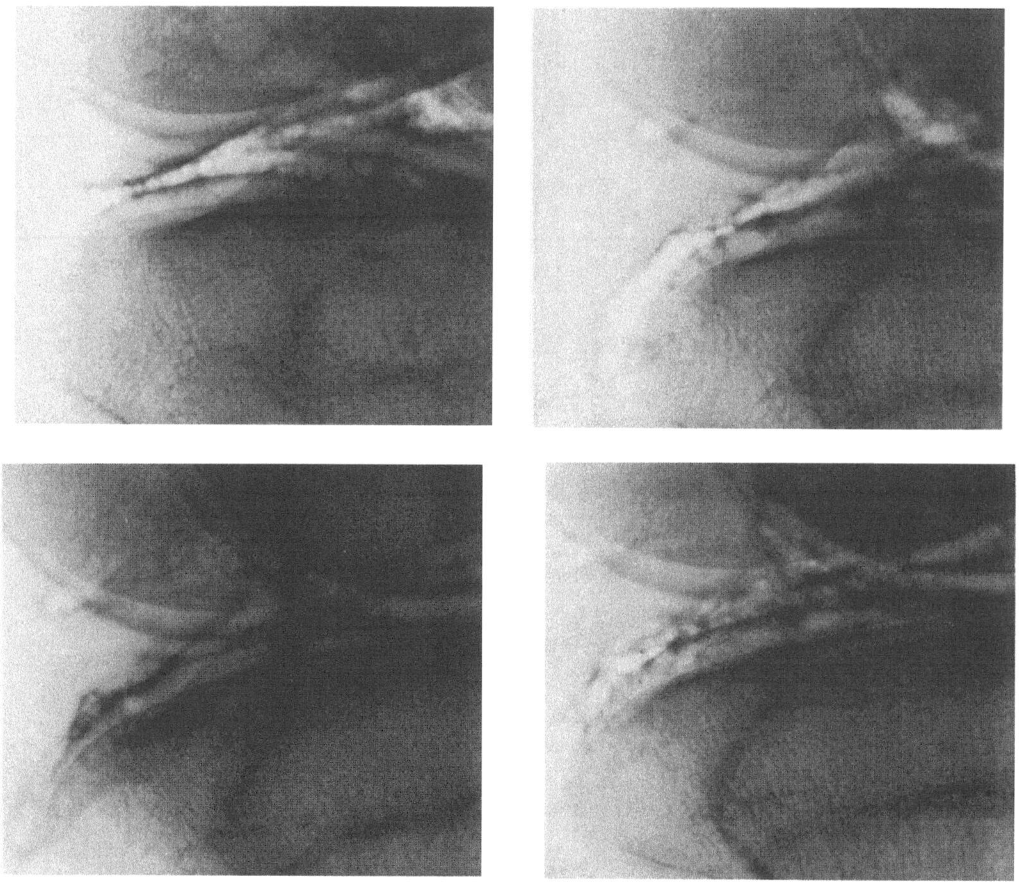

Fig. 27. Details of lateral posterior horn. No visualization of the tendon sheath of the popliteus muscle

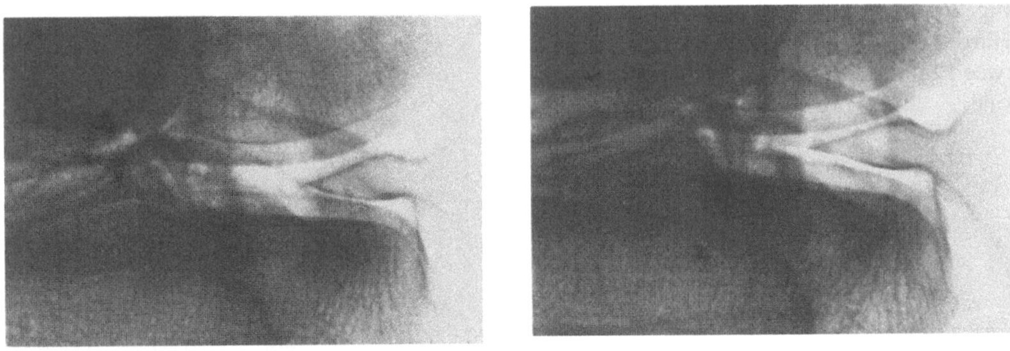

Fig. 28. Lateral posterior horn. No visualization of the tendon sheath of the popliteus muscle. Firm connection between lateral posterior horn and capsule

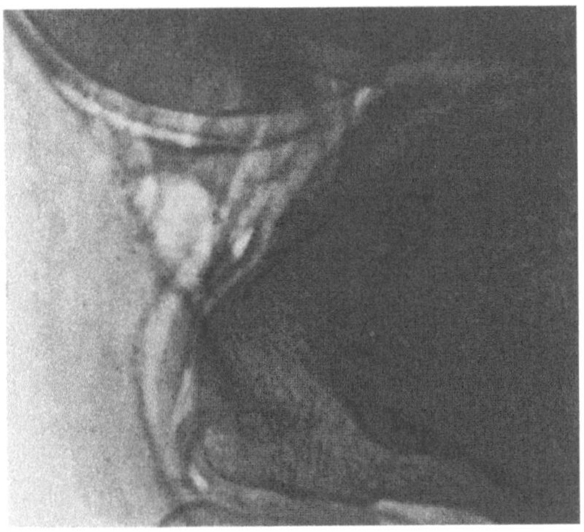

Fig. 29. Communication between the articular cavities of the tibiofemoral and the tibiofibular joint

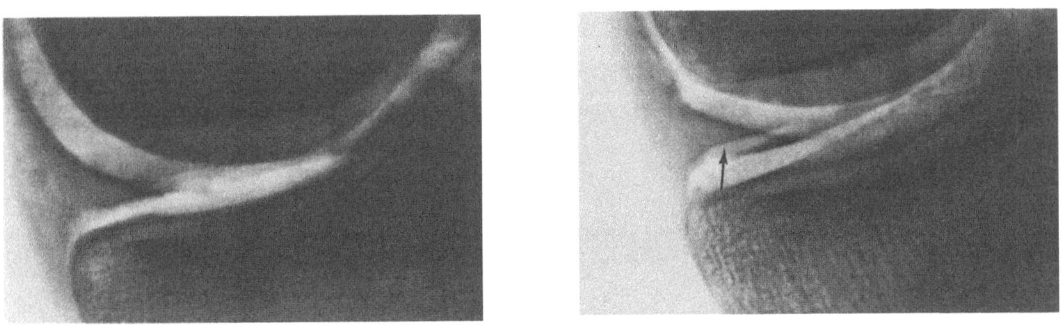

Fig. 30. Medial meniscus. Apparent rupture of the central part, caused by superposition of articular cartilage (*arrow*). No arthroscopic changes

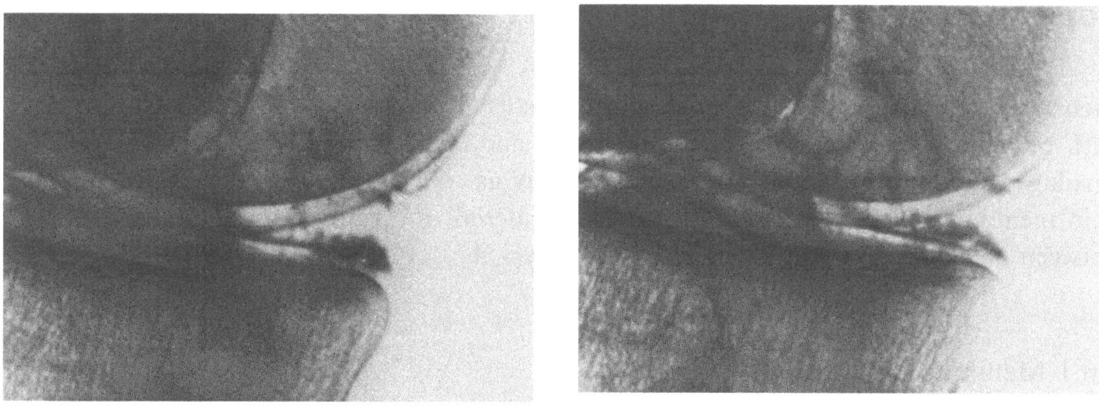

Fig. 31. Normal medial meniscus. Overprojection of free contrast medium in the intra-articular space over the meniscal contour

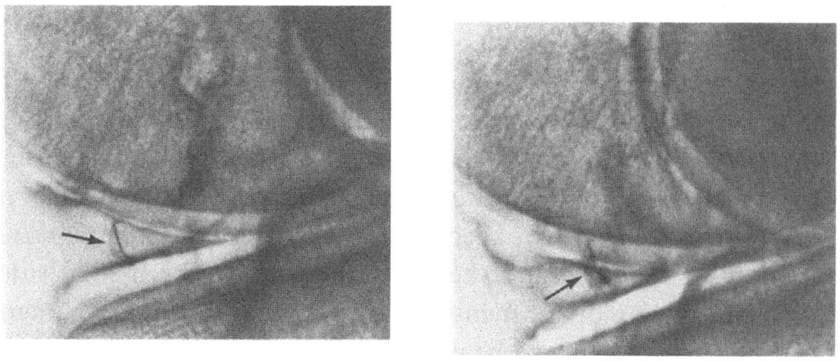

Fig. 32. Apparent rupture of the posterior horn of the medial meniscus, caused by superposition of artefact (*arrow*)

impression caused by superposition of articular cartilage (Fig. 30). On the other hand, overprojection of contrast medium free in the intra-articular space can cause an apparent irregularity of the meniscal contour (Fig. 31). In Fig. 32, a vertical rupture is suggested by superposition of an annular shadow which defines exact description. The description of the normal features of the medial meniscus has already mentioned the possibility of confusion concerning meniscal ruptures, due to depiction of the infrapatellar synovial fold and hypertrophic flocculi of Hoffa's body or synovium. The presence of foam in the intra-articular space rarely poses problems in the diagnosis of meniscal lesions (Fig. 66). However, cartilaginous corpora libera can produce an intra-articular shadow, in which case a meniscal lesion cannot always be excluded with certainty.

3.6 Meniscal Lesions

Meniscal lesions can be found as fresh ruptures or as old ruptures, with or without degeneration of the meniscus and/or articular cartilage. In addition, lesions after meniscectomy as well as discoid meniscus will be discussed. In our case material, the ratio between medial and lateral meniscal lesions was 7:4.

3.6.1 Meniscal Ruptures

The various ruptures to be found in menisci can be divided as schematically indicated in Fig. 33.

3.6.1.1 Tangential Incisure

In the majority of cases, tangential incisures are found on the inferior aspect of the menisci. This is explained by the fact that the menisci rotate passively and synchronously with the rotatory movements of the femoral condyles over the tibial plateau. An extensor movement can keep the meniscus incarcerated between the femoral condyle and the tibial plateau. On the medial side, the firm fixation of the meniscus to capsule and medial ligament causes a tensile force to be exerted on the incarcerated posterior horn, and this can result in incisure. An incisure can be regarded as a beginning of total meniscal rupture (Figs. 33–35). Figure 36 shows an incisure on the superior aspect of the lateral posterior horn. It is usually possible to distinguish a tangential incisure from a recess, but in some cases differentiation is difficult. Figure 37 shows notches on the superior as well as the inferior aspect of the medial posterior horn, both of which could be small incisures. Differentiation from a recess is not always possible by arthrography. Arthroscopic examination of this patient revealed no lesions. Incomplete separation between medial posterior horn and capsule is nearly always based on partial detachment of the medial meniscus (Fig. 38). Figure 39 shows a flaccid medial collateral ligament and a narrow fissure between the superior aspect of the medial meniscus and the capsule. Arthroscopic examination disclosed slight synovial proliferation at this site, and consequently some slight detachment of the medial meniscus is involved (which may have been more marked). Figure 40 illustrates a similar case; there was a small separation between medial posterior horn and capsule; the arthroscopist found no lesions.

Fig. 33. I Tangential incisure. IIa, b and c: Longitudinal rupture (without and with luxation of the detached central part). III Fish mouth rupture. IV Transverse rupture. V Combined rupture

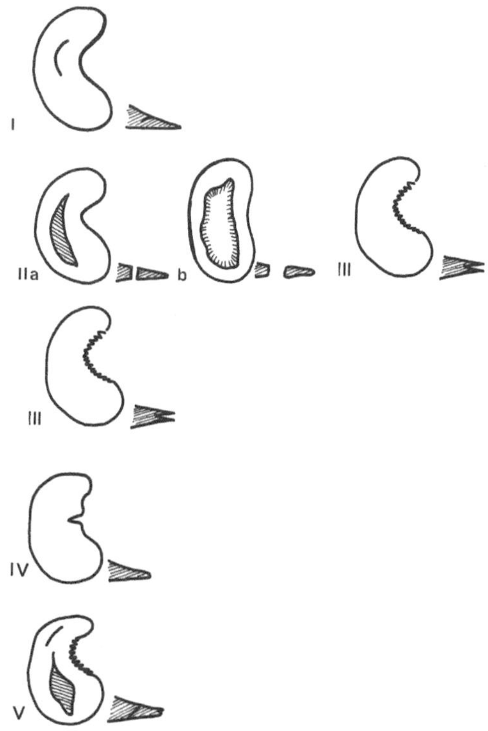

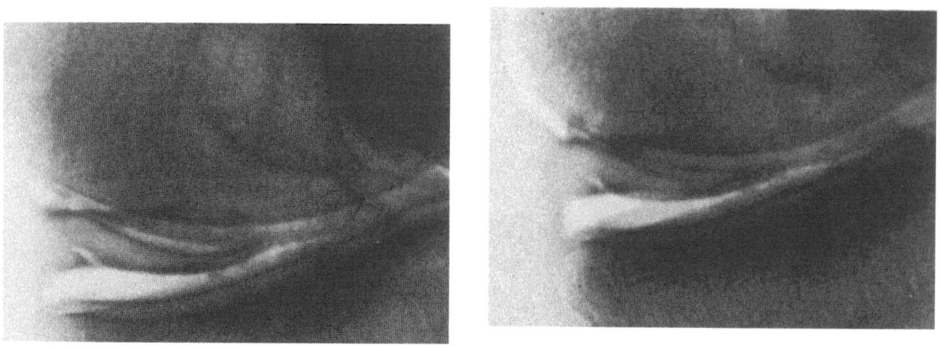

Fig. 34. Posterior horn of medial meniscus. Incisure of the tibial meniscal contour

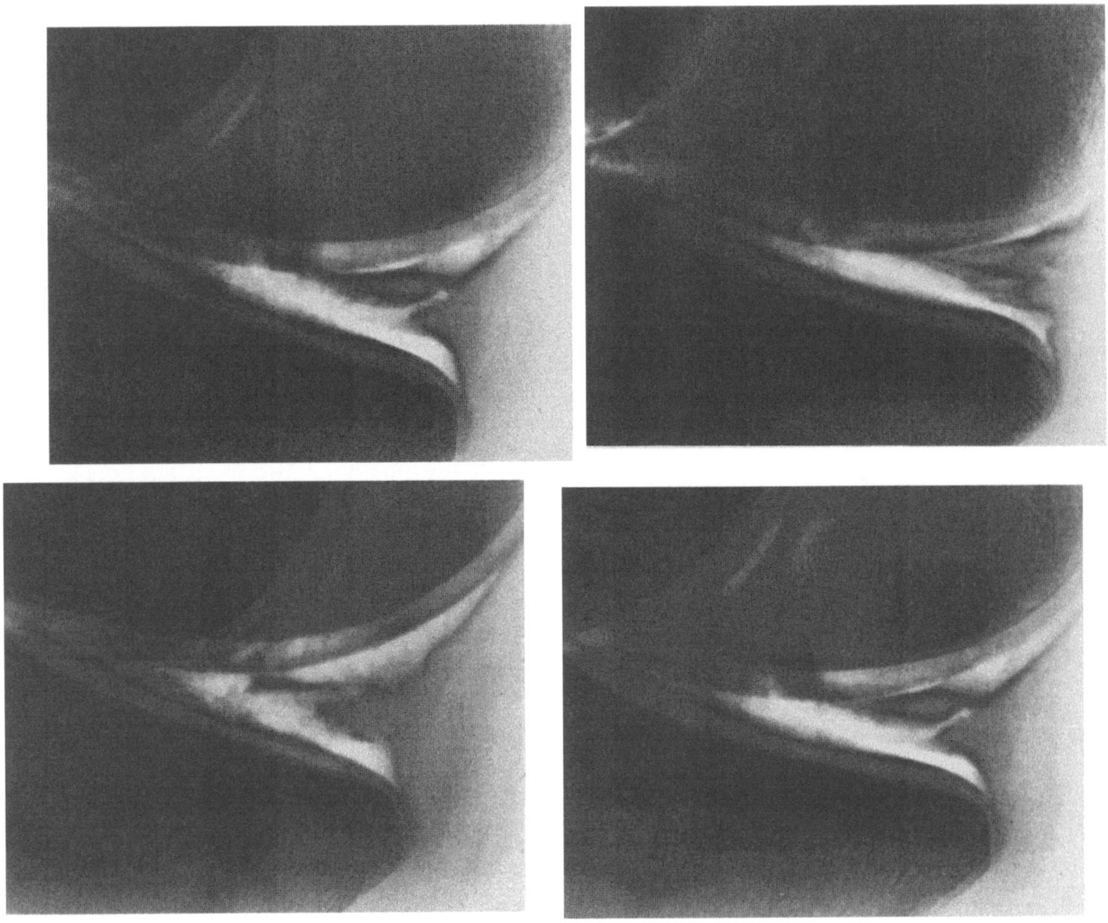

Fig. 35. Projections of the posterior horn of medial meniscus. Deep incisure on the underside of the meniscus

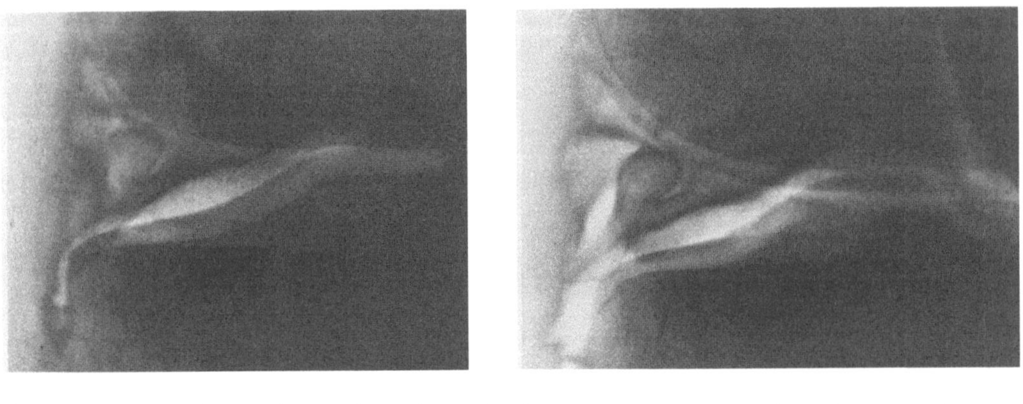

Fig. 36. Posterior horn of lateral meniscus. Incisure on the superior side of the meniscus

Fig. 37. Posterior horn of medial meniscus. Discontinuity between meniscus and capsule on the superior as well as on the inferior side. The former discontinuity is probably a normal recess. The latter can be either a recess or a rupture. No arthroscopic lesions

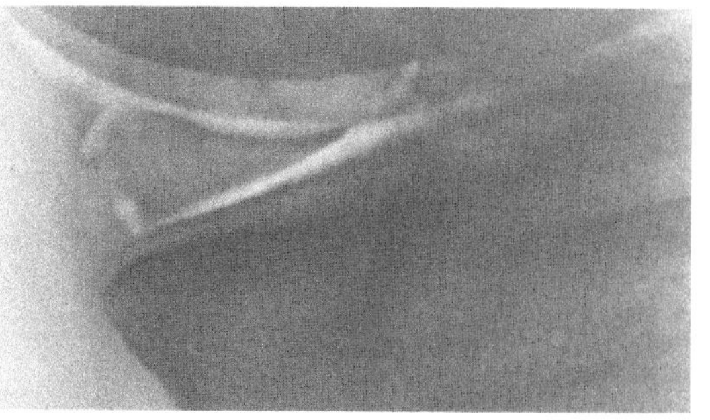

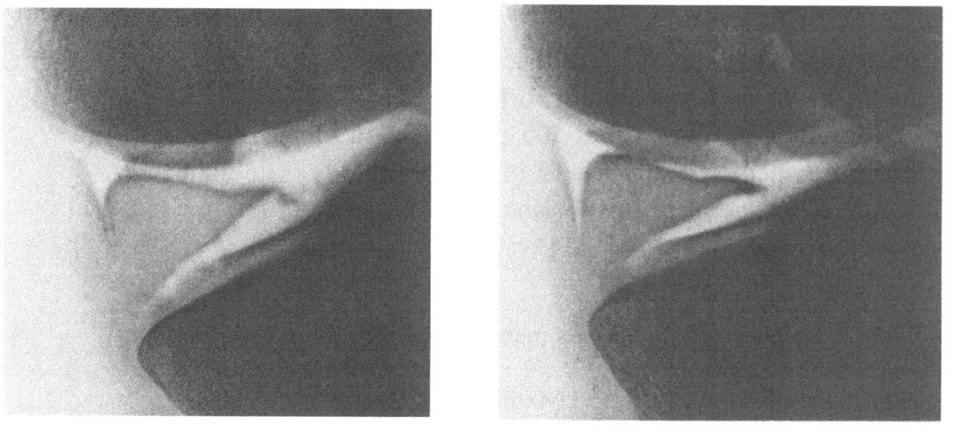

Fig. 38. Posterior horn of medial meniscus. Incomplete separation between medial posterior horn and capsule. Almost certainly partial detachment of the medial meniscus. Mild degeneration of the central margin

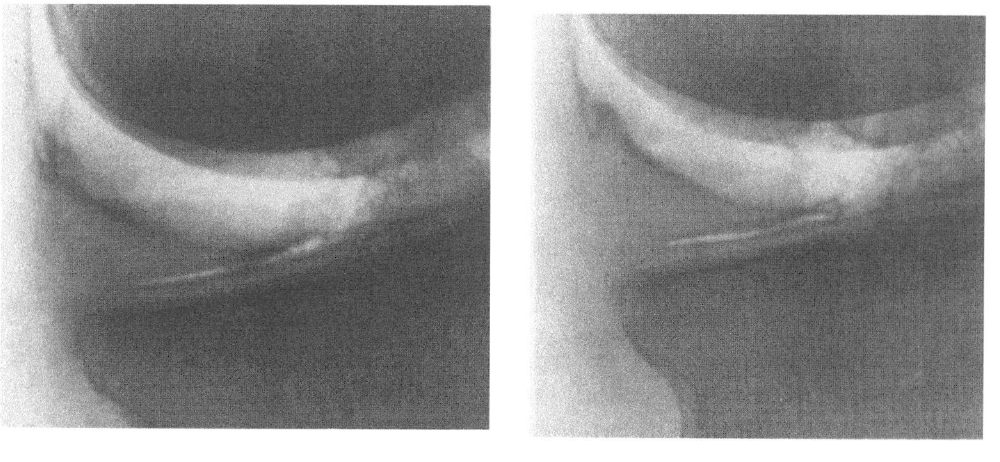

Fig. 39. Central part of medial meniscus. Flaccid medial collateral ligament and small separation between superior side of meniscus and capsule: partial detachment? Arthroscopy: slight synovial proliferation

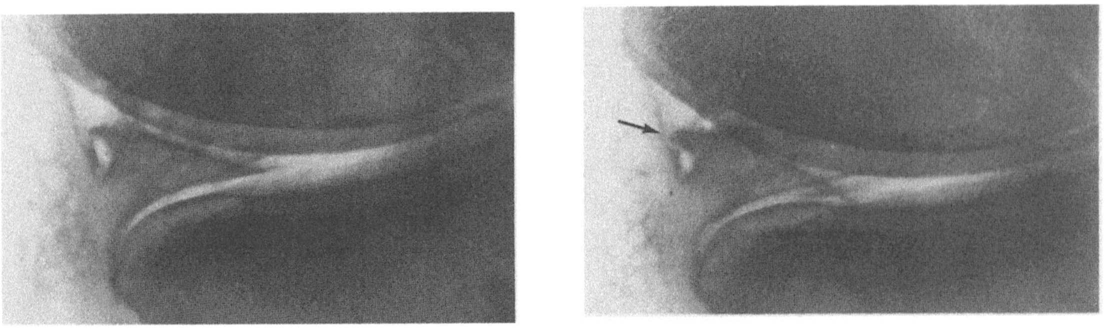

Fig. 40. Medial meniscus. Arthrographic diagnosis: small incisure and synovial reaction (*arrow*). Arthroscopy: no lesions. Conclusion: probably small incisure

Since tangential incisure produces no detached meniscal fragments, lock symptoms are not to be expected.
In a random group of about 500 patients with meniscal lesions, tangential incisures were found in 14% (Table 1). The majority of tangential incisures involve the inferior aspect of the medial meniscus.

Table 1. Incidence of the various meniscal lesions

Types of lesion	Medial meniscus	Lateral meniscus	Total
Tangential incisure	17%	11%	14%
Longitudinal rupture	41%	16%	33%
Fish mouth rupture et al.	4%	9%	6%
Combined rupture	11%	3%	8%
Discoid meniscus	1%	10%	3%
After meniscectomy	20%	32%	25%
Degenerative lesions	6%	19%	11%

3.6.1.2 Longitudinal Ruptures

During examination, sufficient dilatation of the articular cavity should be ensured; this generally facilitates the diagnosis of meniscal lesions considerably (Fig. 84).
A longitudinal rupture can be regarded as an extension of a tangential incisure (Figs. 33 and 41–44). Intercondylar luxation of the detached central part produces rupture type II b as drawn in Fig. 33 (Figs. 45 and 46). This type of rupture is known as bucket-handle rupture. A longitudinal rupture of part of the meniscus can cause partial detachment of the central meniscal

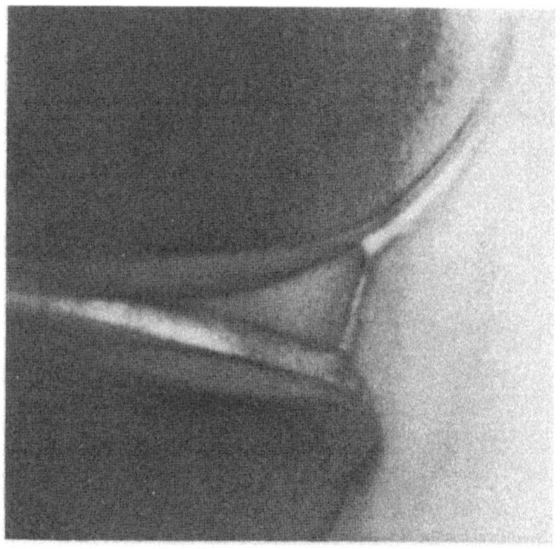

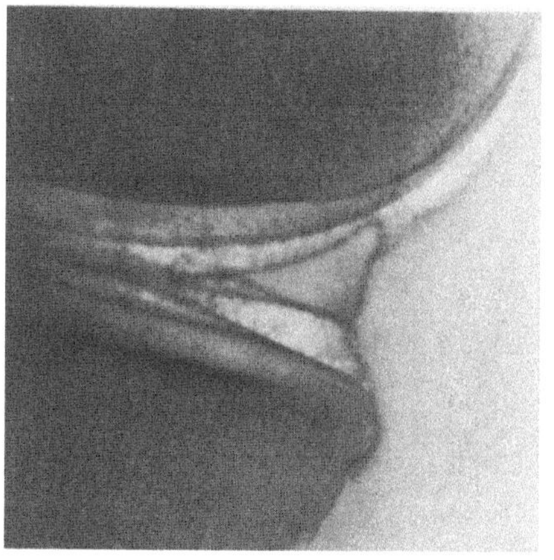

Fig. 41. Medial meniscus with longitudinal rupture

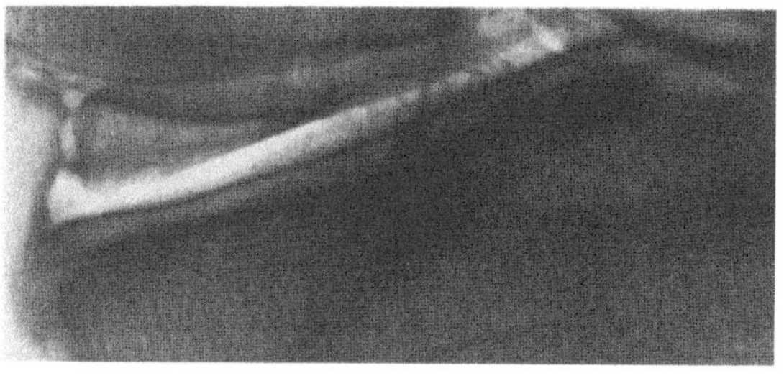

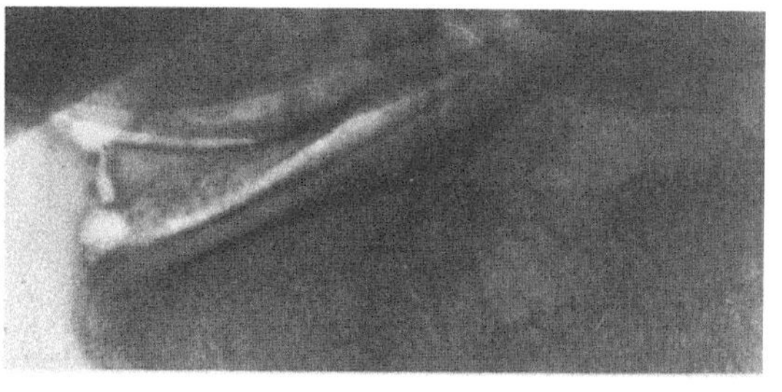

Fig. 42. Posterior horn of medial meniscus. Longitudinal meniscal rupture and unmistakable meniscal lesion. Arthroscopy: no lesions! Conclusion: false negative arthroscopic result

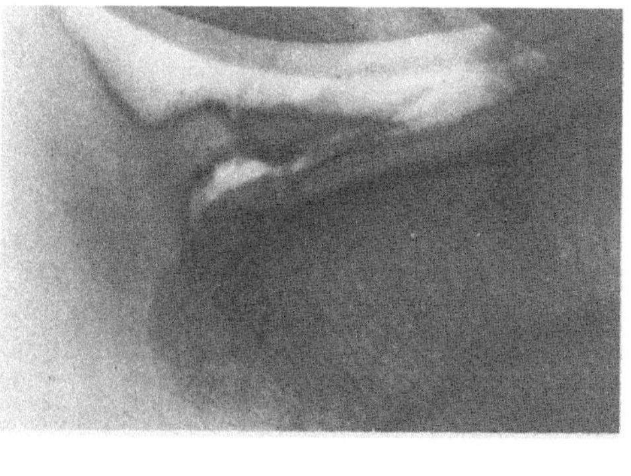

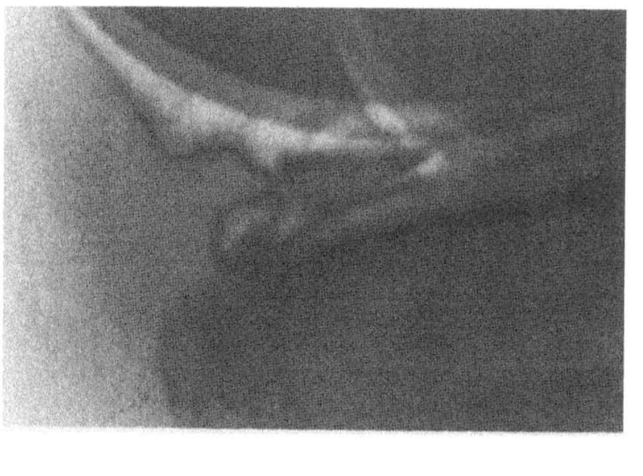

Fig. 43. Posterior horn of medial meniscus. Longitudinal rupture and unmistakable meniscal lesion. Arthroscopy: no lesions! Conclusion: false negative arthroscopic result

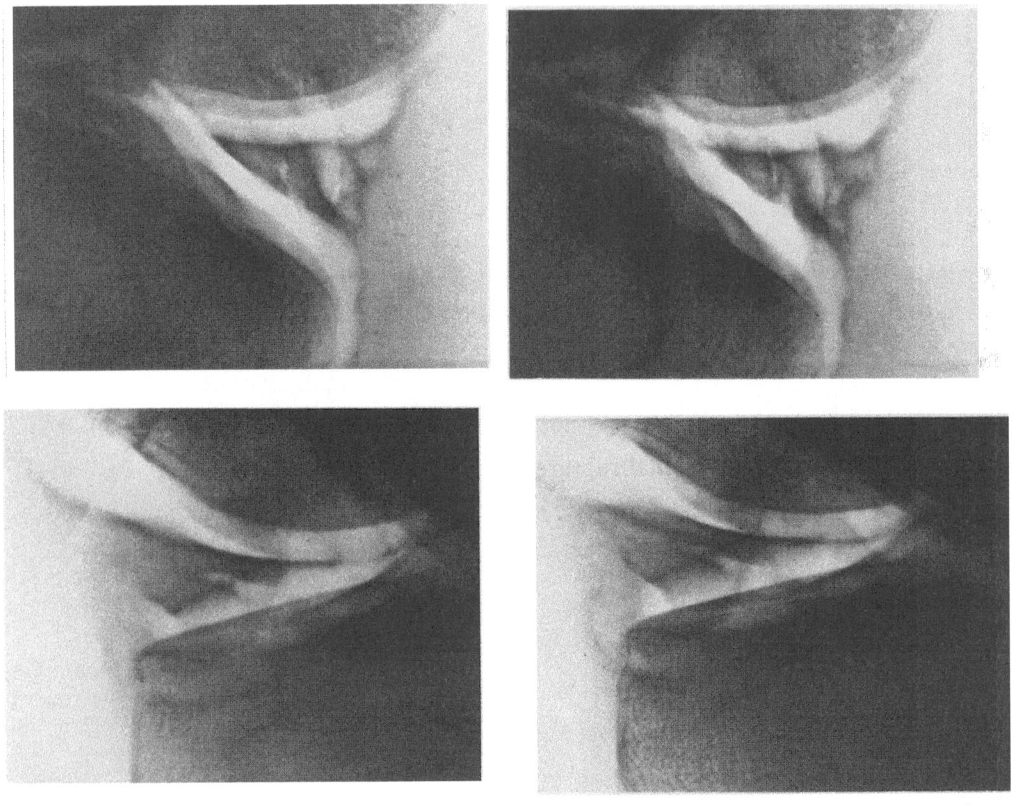

a

b

Fig. 44. (a) Posterior horn of lateral meniscus. Longitudinal rupture of posterior horn central to the tendon sheath of the popliteus muscle. (b) Anterior horn of lateral meniscus. Incisure on the inferior side of the meniscus

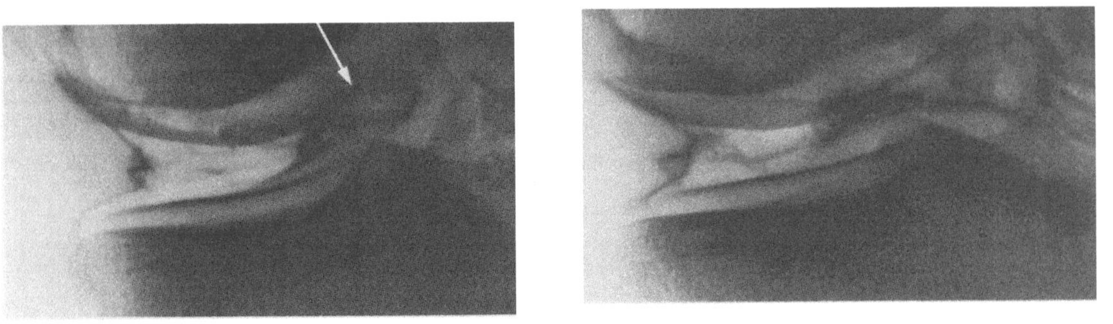

Fig. 45. Central part of medial meniscus. Rupture type II b. Total rupture and luxation of the detached part of the meniscus (*arrow*). Bucket-handle rupture

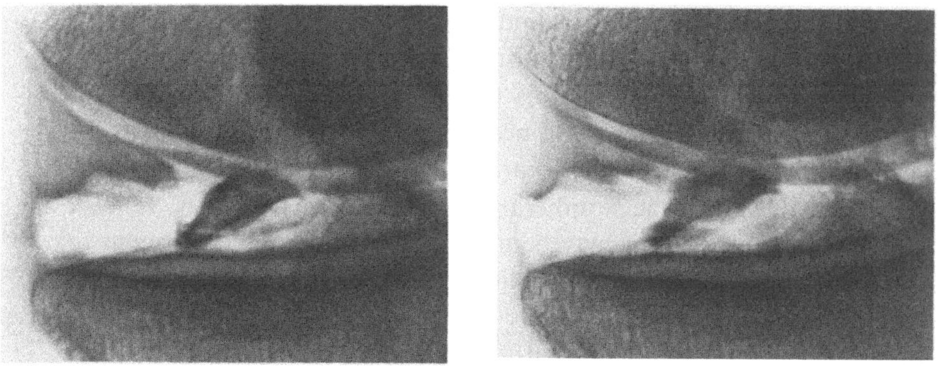

Fig. 46. Medial meniscus. Bucket-handle rupture. Clearly visible detached part of meniscus and frayed delimitation of peripheral stump

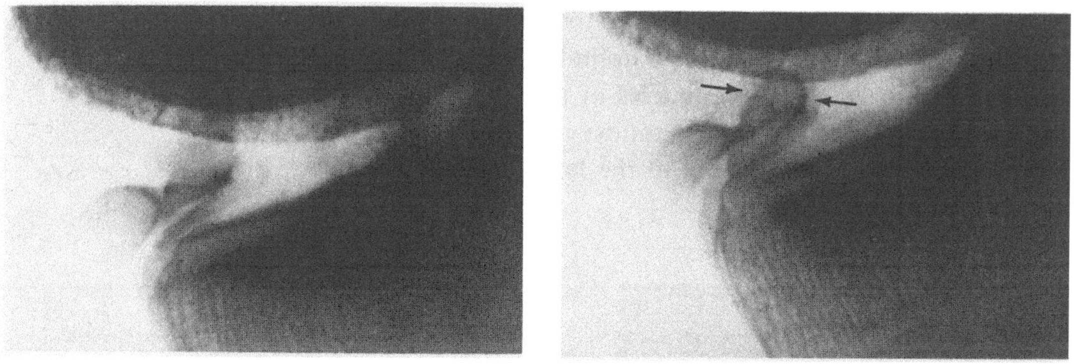

Fig. 47. Medial meniscus. Rupture type IIc. Part of the central margin of the meniscus is detached. The detached part remains in contact with the anterior or the posterior horn and is projected obliquely above the peripheral meniscal remnant (*arrows*)

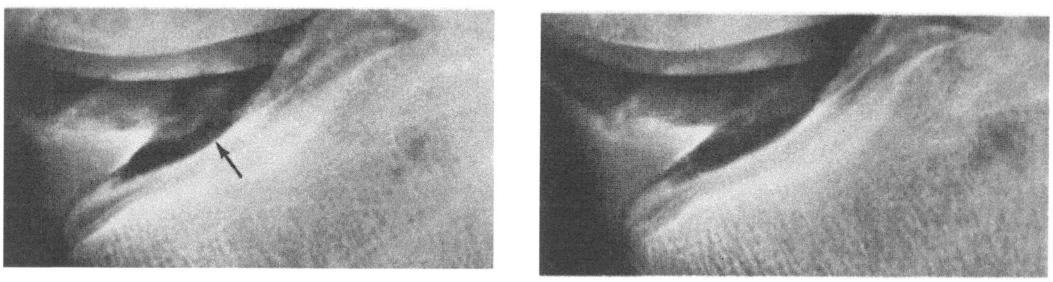

Fig. 48. Medial meniscus. Rupture type IIc. Partly detached central meniscal margin (*arrow*). Verification by arthroscopy

margin, the detached part remaining in contact with the anterior or the posterior horn of the meniscus (Figs. 47 and 48). Particularly in meniscal ruptures of this type (IIc), exact depiction of the central margin is important, because this often shows lesions. The usually reversed, partly separated portion of the meniscus is often visible above the peripheral part of the meniscus (Figs. 15 and 47). In some cases it may be necessary to differentiate from synovial hypertrophy or a mobile flocculus of Hoffa's body (Fig. 150).
Longitudinal ruptures of types IIa, IIb, and IIc were found in 33% of meniscal lesions (Table 1). As expected, the medial meniscus was involved in the majority of cases (41%).

3.6.1.3 Fish Mouth Ruptures

In these cases a horizontal rupture of the meniscus causes the central margin to assume the shape of an open fish mouth by arthrography (Figs. 49–51). According to Smillie (1975), fish mouth ruptures are most likely to be found in degenerated menisci. In the majority of cases ruptures of this type involve the lateral meniscus (Table 1). In this context it is to be noted that transverse ruptures, found mainly in the lateral meniscus, have been included in this category.

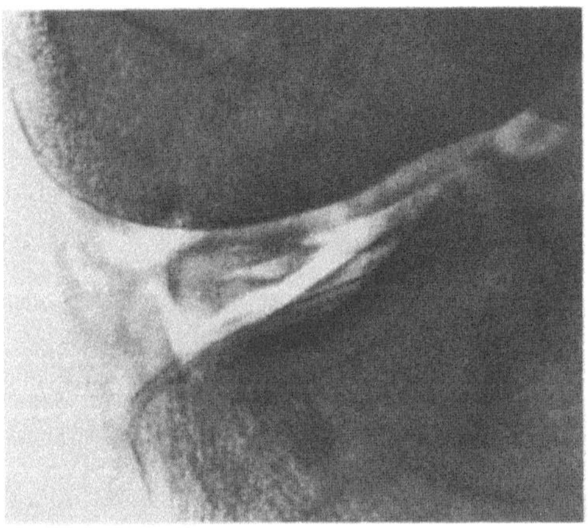

Fig. 49. Lateral meniscus. Fish mouth rupture in central part

3.6.1.4 Transverse Ruptures

These ruptures, indicated as type IV in Fig. 33 and found mainly in the lateral meniscus, are rarely identifiable as such by ar-

Fig. 50. Lateral meniscus. Fish mouth rupture

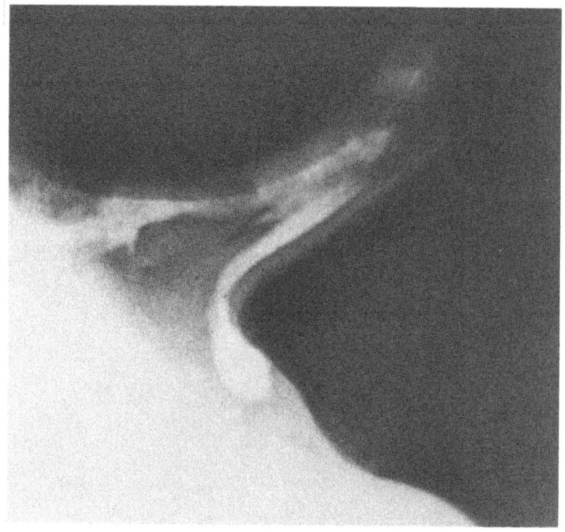

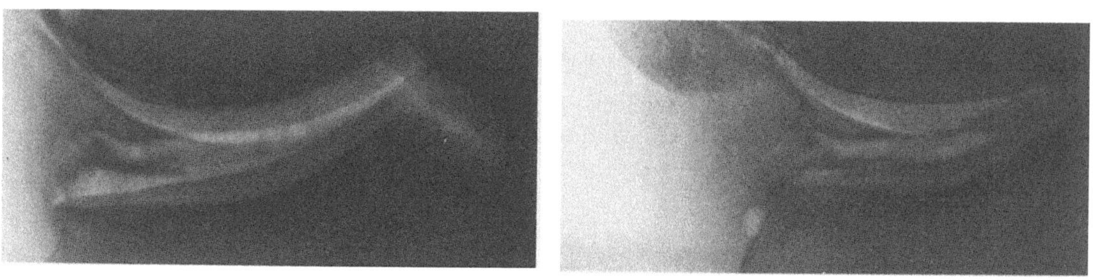

Fig. 51. Lateral meniscus. Fish mouth rupture. Arthroscopy: corroboration

thrography. At best, the central margin of the meniscus is slightly irregular, which may raise suspicion that a rupture exists at this site. For this reason, transverse ruptures have not been included in Table 1 as a separate category. Menisci with a less regular central margin possibly due to transverse rupture, were added to the fish mouth ruptures.

3.6.1.5 Combined Ruptures

This category includes all ruptures which cannot be brought under a single heading but involve a combination of rupture types already discussed (Figs. 52 and 53). Combined ruptures account for 8% of all meniscal lesions listed in Table 1; in most cases the medial meniscus was involved.

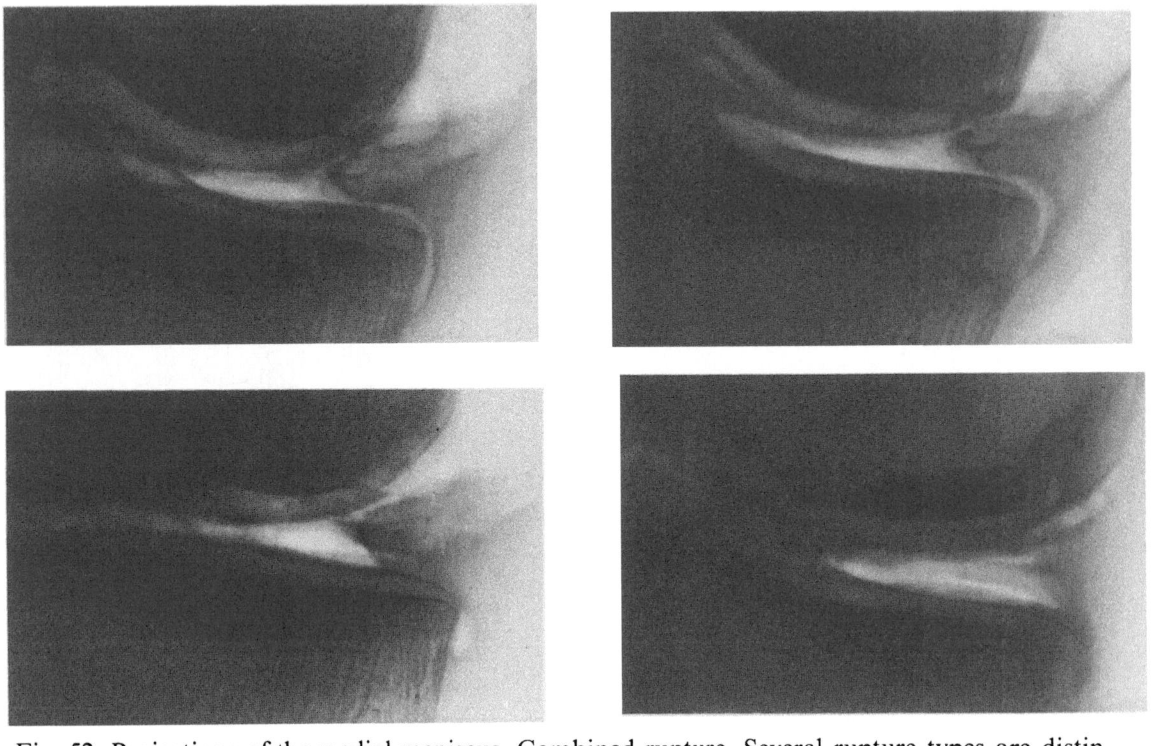

Fig. 52. Projections of the medial meniscus. Combined rupture. Several rupture types are distinguishable: incisure, fish mouth rupture and longitudinal rupture. Luxation of a detached part of the meniscus

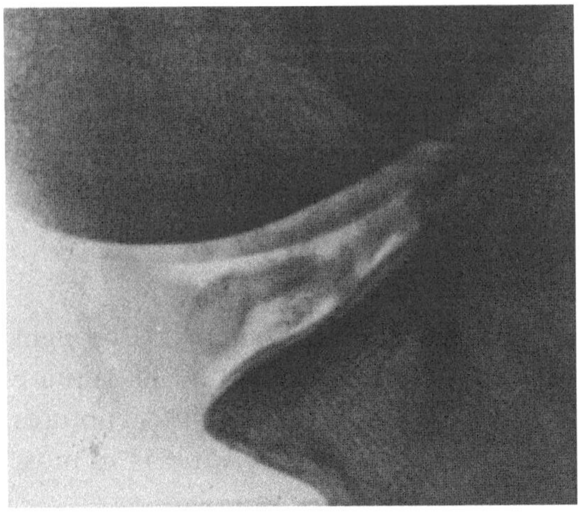

Fig. 53. Posterior horn of medial meniscus. Combined rupture, the meniscus showing incisure, longitudinal rupture with detached fragment, and secondary degeneration

3.6.2. Types of Discoid Meniscus

In embryos of 30–35 mm length, the tibial plateau is separated from the femoral condyles by plates of mesenchymal tissue that, at an embryo length of 38–45 mm, become detached from femur and tibial head. Before the fifth embryonic month, these cartilaginous tissue plates are believed to be so far resorbed in the central portion that the normal circular form of the meniscus emerges (Smillie, 1951, 1975; Baumgartl, 1964). The above-mentioned cartilage discs between femur and tibia are normally present in rats and birds.

According to Kaplan (1955, 1957) a discoid meniscus results from increased mobility mainly of the lateral posterior horn, which consequently is repeatedly under considerable stress. This hypothesis is probably untenable.

The following types of discoid meniscus are distinguished (Fig. 54).

Type A: An entirely disc-shaped meniscus extending almost to the intercondylar eminence

Type B: With the central margin showing a slightly concave delimitation

Type C: Characterized by a very large posterior horn

Type D: Characterized by a very large anterior horn

Type E: An annular type of meniscus, with a central open space

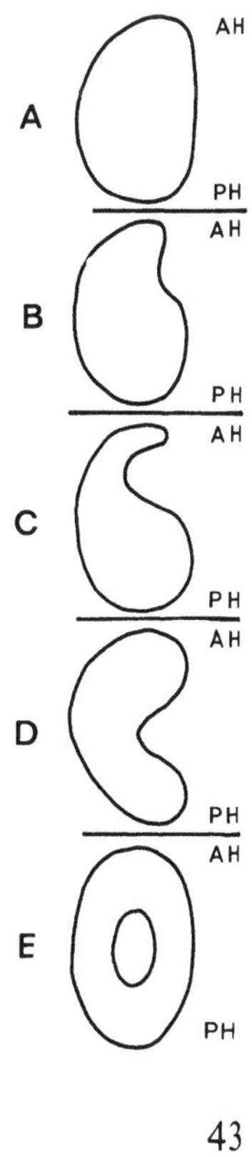

Fig. 54. Types of discoid meniscus: Type A: complete discoid meniscus, Type B: slightly concave delimitation of central margin, Type C and D: large posterior horn, anterior horn, respectively, caused by excentric deep concave central margin, Type E: annular meniscus with central opening

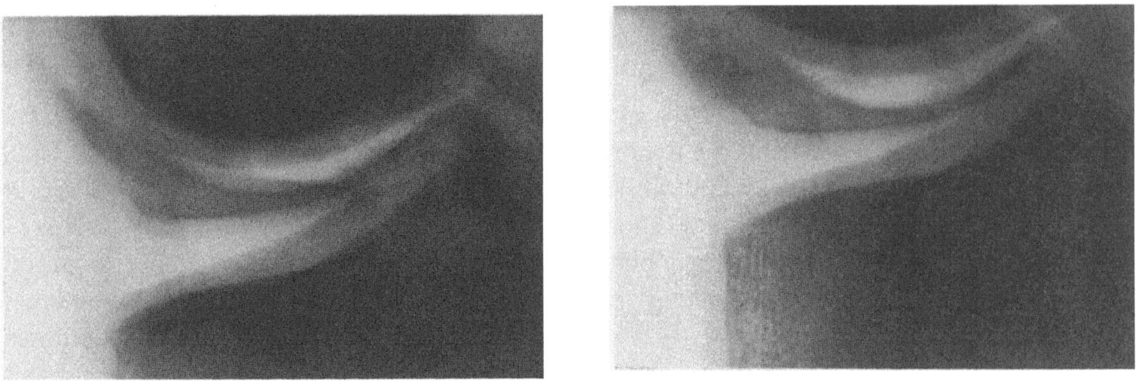

Fig. 55. Discoid lateral meniscus, type A

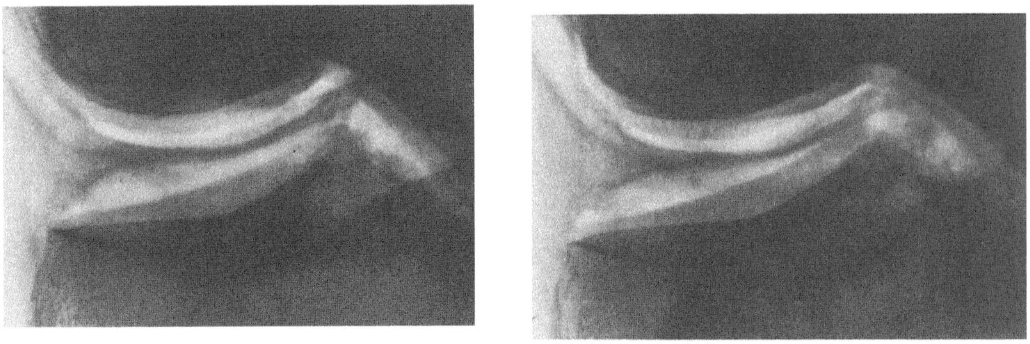

Fig. 56. Discoid lateral meniscus, type A

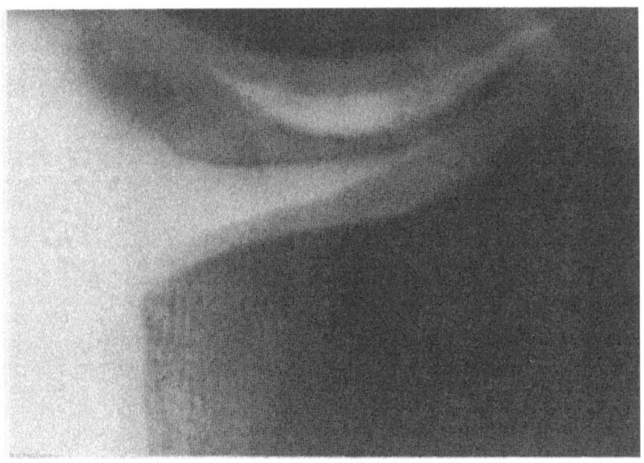

Fig. 57. Discoid lateral meniscus, type A

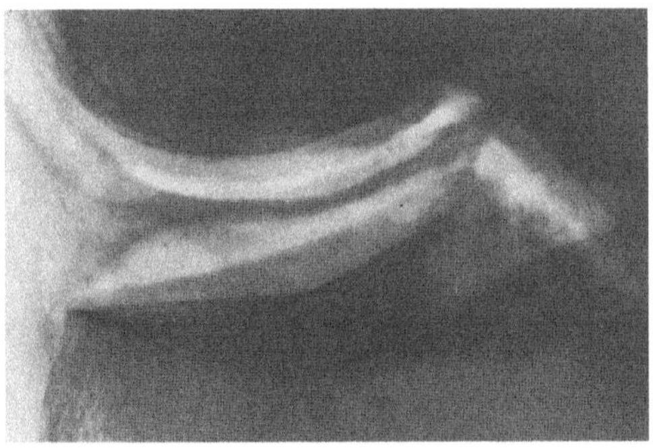

Fig. 58. Discoid medial meniscus. Partial superposition of the meniscus on the tibial plateau

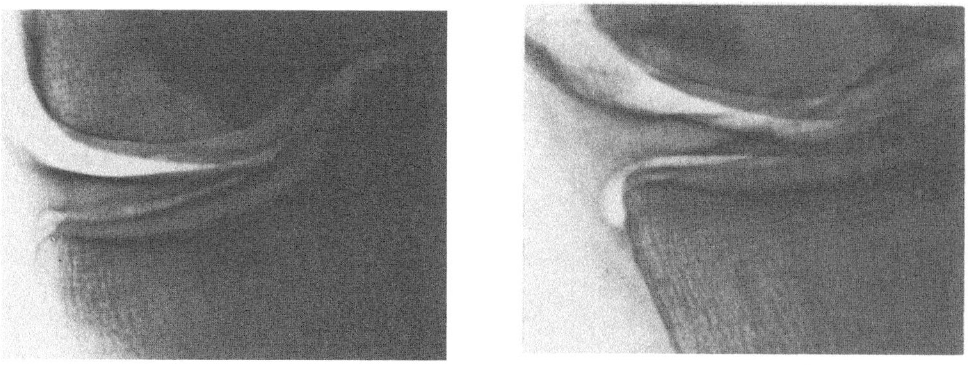

Fig. 59. Discoid medial meniscus, type D. The anterior horn in particular extends far centrally

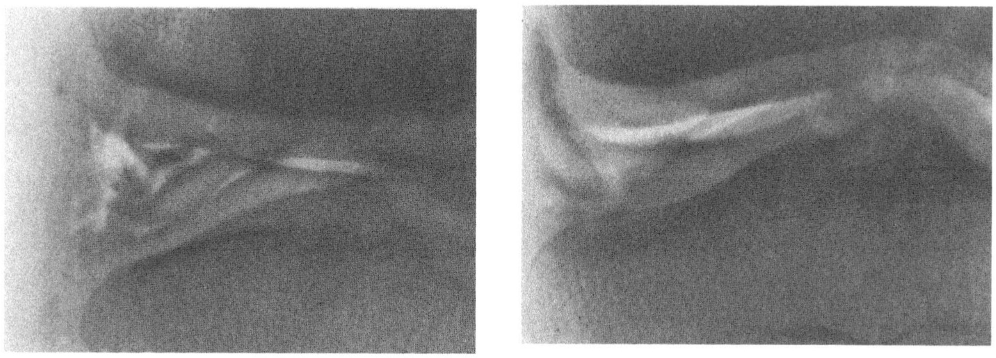

Fig. 60. Male, age 10. Projections of the lateral meniscus. Ruptured discoid lateral meniscus. Arthroscopy: corroboration

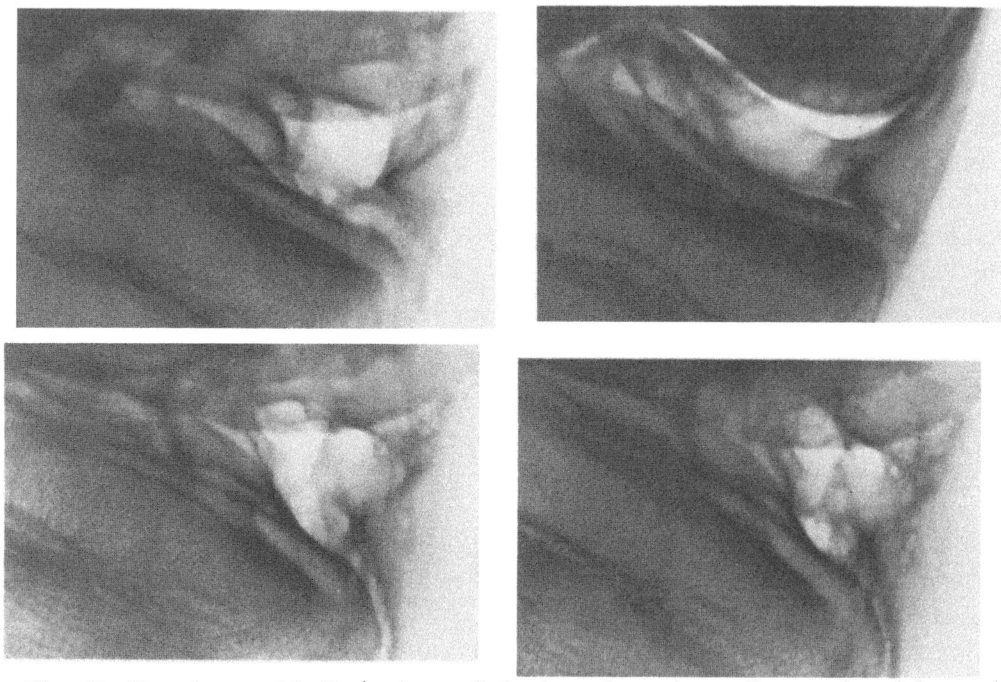

Fig. 61. Female, age 10. Projections of the lateral meniscus. Ruptured and luxated discoid lateral meniscus. Arthroscopy: corroboration

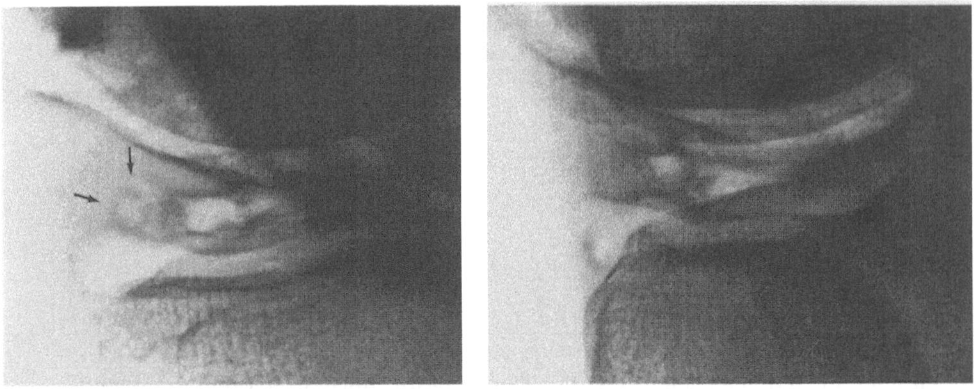

Fig. 62. Male, age 51. Projections of the lateral meniscus. Ruptured and degenerated discoid lateral meniscus. Degenerative cavities in the meniscus communicate with the articular cavity (*arrows*)

A discoid meniscus can give rise to symptoms of incarceration and ruptures. The recurrent incarcerations cause degenerative lesions. A meniscal lesion during the first decade of life is not infrequently based on a discoid meniscus. Most types of discoid meniscus are lateral menisci. Double contrast arthrography can readily demonstrate a discoid meniscus. Type A in intact condition is visible on arthrograms as a broad cartilage plate extending into the center of the joint (Figs. 55–57).
A discoid meniscus is usually lateral, but may occasionally be medial. Smillie (1975) studied 8,000 meniscal lesions and found 375 lateral and only 5 medial discoid menisci (Figs. 58 and 59).
Figures 60 and 61 show ruptured lateral discoid menisci found in two 10-year-old children. Figure 62 shows a markedly abnormal meniscal shape resulting from rupture and degeneration of a lateral discoid meniscus. Discoid menisci were found in 3% of the random group of successively registered meniscal lesions listed in Table 1.

3.6.3 Degeneration of Meniscal Cartilage

3.6.3.1 Primary Degeneration (Including Cystic Degeneration)

Degeneration is regarded as a biologic reaction of the meniscus to compressive lesions and nutritional disorders. Bonnin (1953) maintained that cystic meniscal degeneration is of traumatic origin in 30% of cases; a similar percentage is nontraumatic, and another 30% results from recurrent microtraumata.
Particularly in individuals whose work involves much kneeling

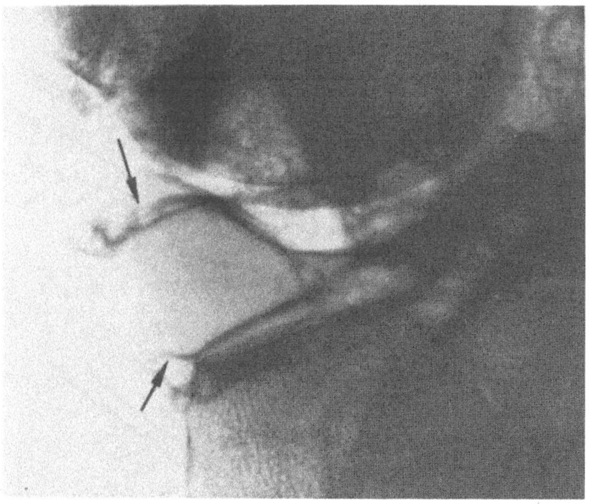

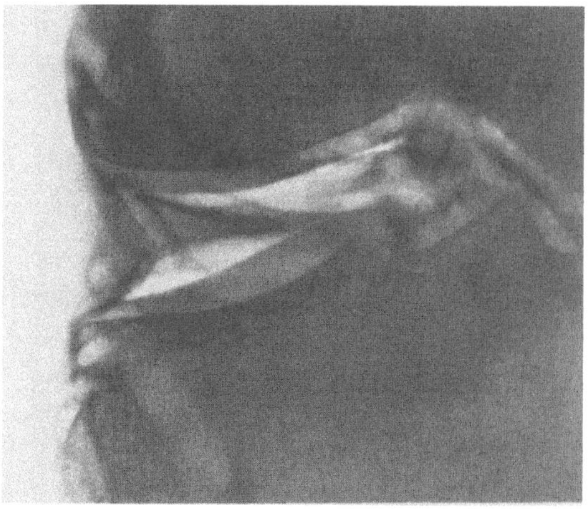

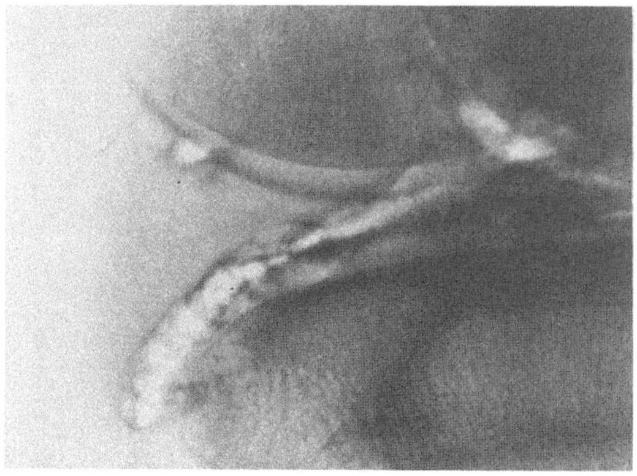

Fig. 63. Projections of the lateral meniscus. Cystic degeneration. The meniscus shows unmistakable peripheral thickening especially in the anterior horn (*arrows*). The contours being intact

or squatting, e.g., miners, the knee joints are subject to excessive stress. The first sign of physiologic degeneration is the presence of finely dispersed fat accumulations in the cytoplasm of the cartilage cells and liquefaction of the intercellular substance (Ricklin et al., 1964, 1971). Later, fatty degeneration is also observed in the intercellular substance, although true tissue lesions are not yet conspicuous. The changes are initially found especially in the superficial parts of the meniscus, but later also in deeper parts. Gradual progression of the degenerative process leads to the formation of larger foci of fatty degeneration and circumscribed necrosis of cartilage. In such cases the regular, smooth meniscal surface assumes a spotted yellowish aspect, while at the same time small incisures and fissures are visible.

Apart from this more diffuse degeneration of meniscal cartilage, there is localized cystic degeneration which usually affects the lateral meniscus. In this condition, also known as meniscal ganglion, there is local thickening of the meniscus, caused by a

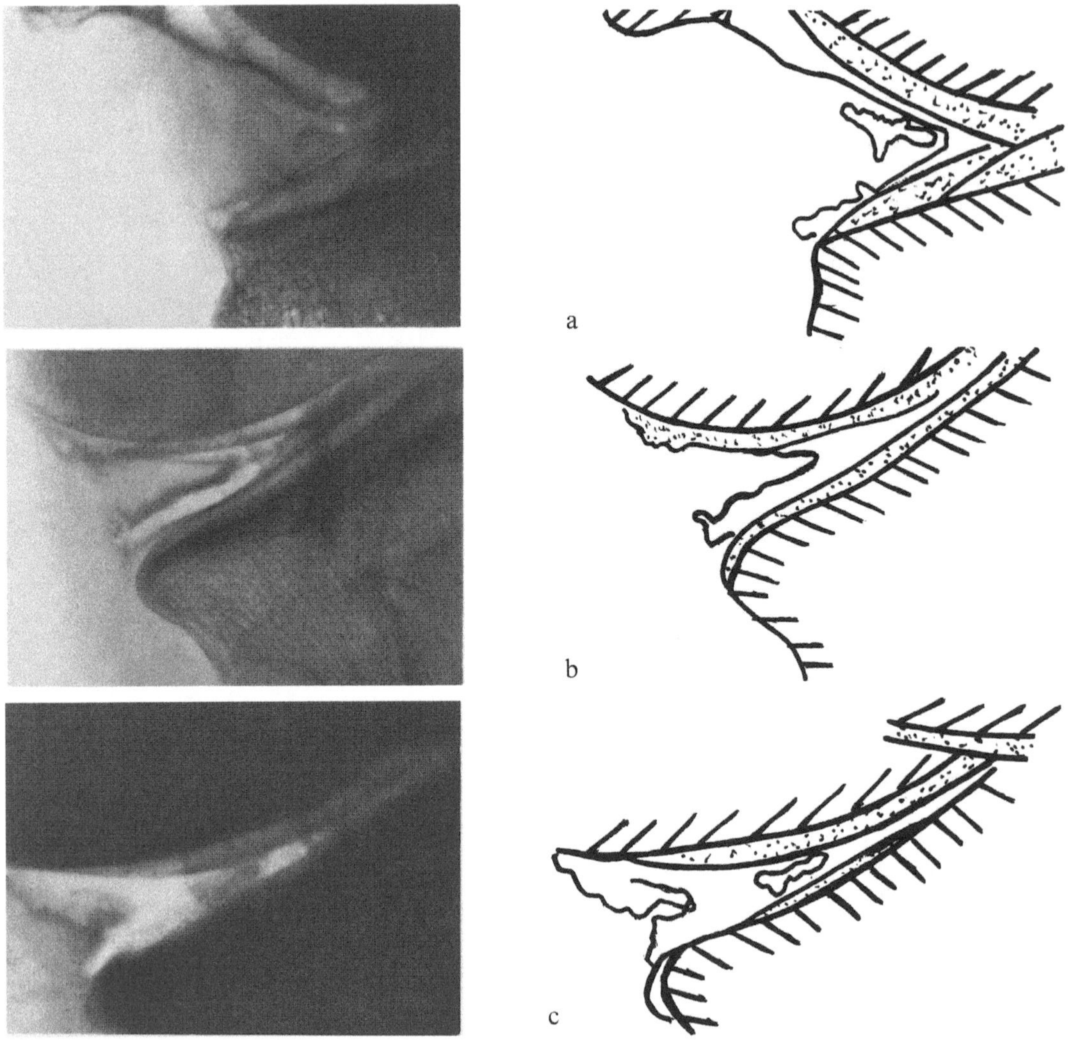

Fig. 64a–c. Degenerative lesions of the meniscus. (a) Cystic degeneration. The degenerative defect communicates with the intra-articular space and is clearly visible. (b) Superficial primary degeneration. Irregular contours of the meniscus. (c) Secondary degeneration of the peripheral meniscal stump with detached fragment and the cartilage of the tibial plateau

multilocular cystic process filled with gelatinous fluid. Evidently, these degenerative processes can gravely undermine the firmness of the menisci, and traumatic injuries are therefore more likely to cause ruptures. Cystic degeneration mostly involves the anterior horn and midportion of the lateral meniscus. In the simplest case; the meniscus is clearly thicker, especially at the periphery, while its contours are intact (Fig. 63). When the degenerative cavities communicate with the articular cavity, both these cavities and their communications with the articular cavity can be visualized by the contrast medium (Fig. 64a).

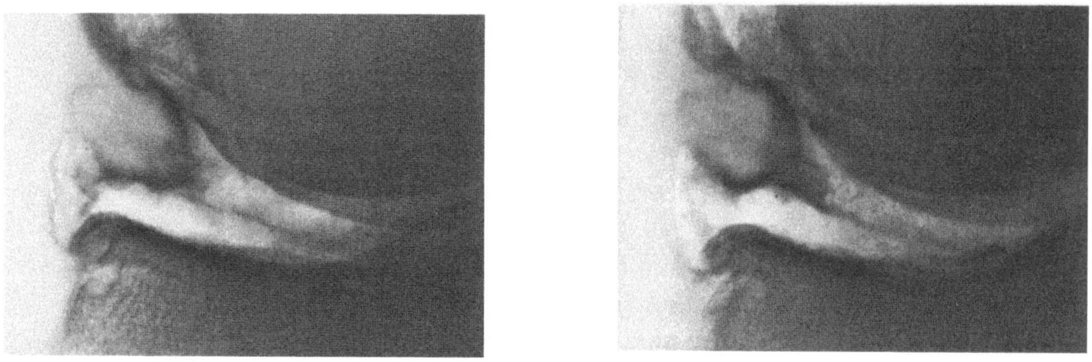

Fig. 65. Lateral meniscus. Cystic degeneration with degenerated contours of the meniscus. Degenerative lesion of the tibial cartilage

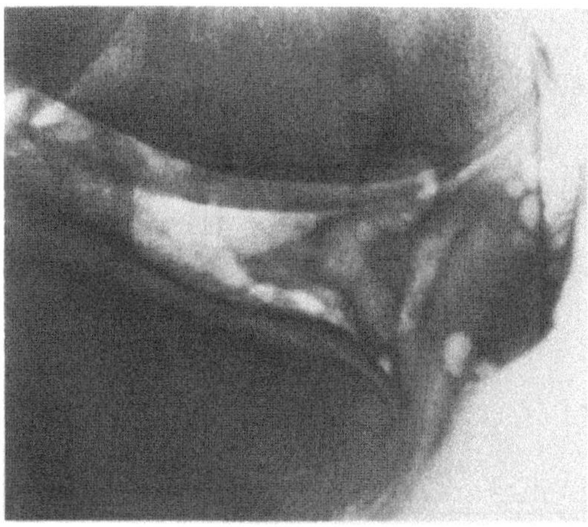

Fig. 66. Posterior horn of lateral meniscus. Intra-articular foam formation. Cystic degeneration of the lateral meniscus with incisures and secondary degeneration at the central margin

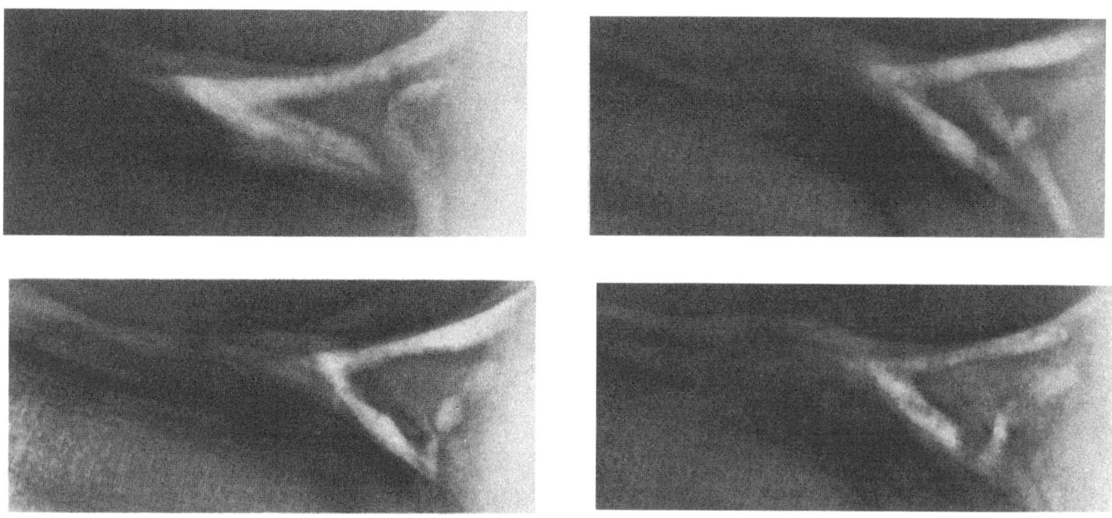

Fig. 67. Projections of the posterior horn of lateral meniscus. Cystic degeneration associated with secondary meniscal degeneration, blunt central margin, and degenerative lesion of the femoral cartilage

In that case the thickened, cystically degenerated meniscus can show a foamy appearance within its contours. The thickened, partly degenerated and already locally divided menisci can of course be damaged by relatively slight injuries (Figs. 65–67). Degenerative meniscal lesions are regularly associated with wasting of the tibial plateau; small peripheral proliferations can also occur (Jonasch, 1960).

Noncystic, more superficial primary degeneration is radiologically visible as irregularity of meniscal contours. Through the uneven cartilage surface, positive contrast medium passes into the superficial layers of the meniscus so that a slightly denser zone of delimitation becomes visible (Fig. 64b). These changes are usually most conspicuous in the thin central part of the meniscus. Menisci thus degenerated can likewise rupture in response to relatively slight injuries.

In knee joints with weak ligaments, degenerative changes can also develop due to excessive movement within the joint. Moreover, small fragments of the menisci can become detached in the synovia. In these cases, histologic examination reveals homogenization of the ground substance, destruction of the fibrous structure, and the presence of necrotic cartilage areas.

3.6.3.2 Secondary Degeneration

It is not always possible to distinguish primary degeneration with meniscal rupture from primary rupture with secondary degeneration of meniscal fragments. In the case of meniscal rupture, the secondary degenerative changes are often localized around

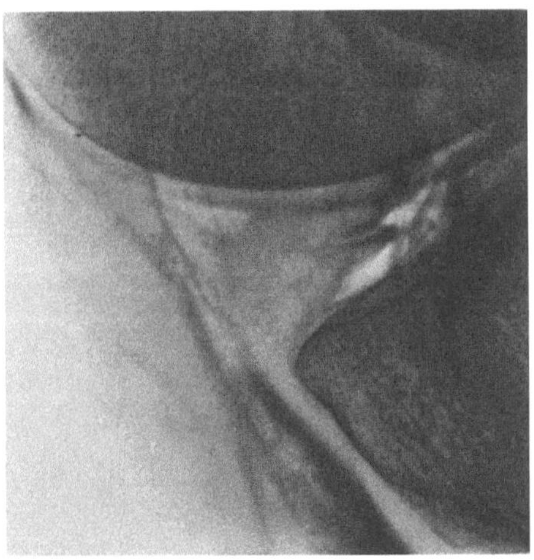

Fig. 68. Posterior horn of lateral meniscus. Fish mouth rupture and secondary degeneration of meniscal cartilage, particularly near the rupture

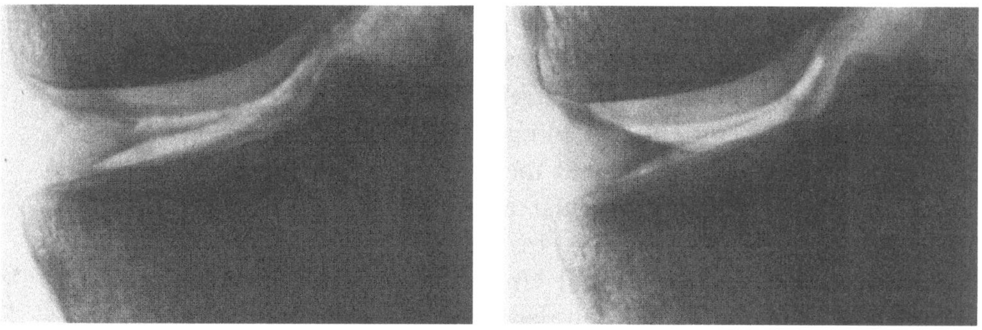

Fig. 69. Central part of medial meniscus. Incisure and secondary degeneration of meniscal cartilage in the immediate vicinity of the incisure

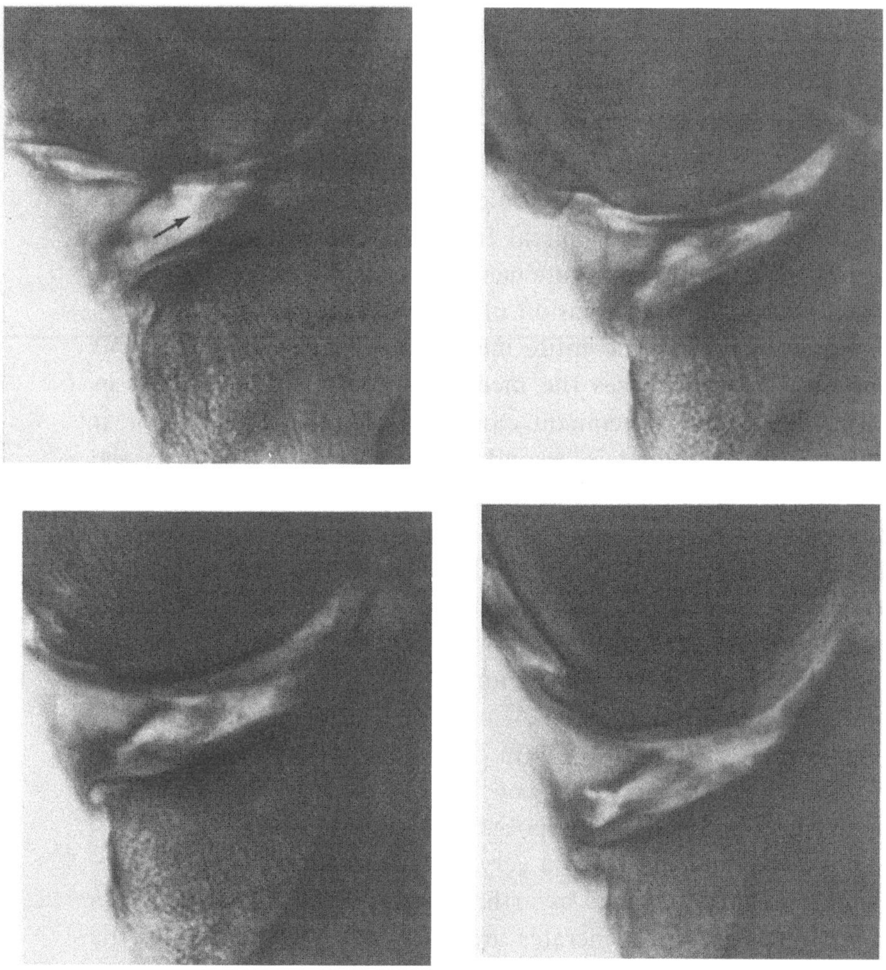

Fig. 70. Projections of the medial meniscus. Old meniscal rupture with detached meniscal fragments (*arrow*); degeneration of articular cartilage and hook formation. Arthrosis deformans

the rupture (Figs. 68 and 69). A central ruptured meniscal fragment, if not removed, assumes increased intra-articular mobility after some considerable time. Recurrent incarceration then gives rise to rapid degeneration. Flattening of the meniscal fragment is often observed. The peripheral meniscal fragment is usually blunt and its contours are irregular and imbibed with contrast medium (Fig. 64c; also Fig. 53). In the case of long-standing meniscal ruptures, the central fragment can disintegrate completely, so that in addition to degeneration of the peripheral meniscal fragment, lesions of the articular cartilage occur. The result is degeneration and unmistakable arthrosis with formation of exostoses (Fig. 70; also Fig. 169).

For the insurance medical officer the distinction between primary degeneration with secondary rupture and primary rupture with secondary degeneration is important. However, it is not always possible to make this distinction.

3.6.4 State After Meniscectomy

There is no agreement on the question whether after meniscal rupture the entire meniscus should be excised or whether removal of only the detached meniscal fragment ensures a good result (cf. p. 138). Unless a separate incision is made behind the medial collateral ligament in excision of a medial meniscus, it is rarely possible to remove the entire meniscus through a more ventral incision. In these cases the medial posterior horn remains in situ. This meniscal remnant can already have ruptured, or it can become ruptured in second instance (Fig. 76). If only the centrally luxated part of the meniscus is removed, the peripheral fragment with its irregular central margin remains in situ. Degenerative changes are frequently observed in this central margin (Debnam and Staple, 1974). If the entire meniscus is excised, then fibrous regeneration starts from the capsule. Radin and Bryan (1970) took an arthrogram in the operating room immediately after meniscectomy. After 6 weeks, regenerates were arthrographically demonstrable in 72% of the patients who had been forbidden to do any lifting and in 39% of those on whom this restriction had not been imposed.

The regenerates consist of a very solid triangular fibrous wedge, which is sharply defined by arthrography (Figs. 71–73). Characteristic feature of regenerates are the regular contours and the triangular shape, which resembles an equilateral triangle, the base and the two rising sides, all roughly equal (2–7 mm). Regenerates rarely show any pathology.

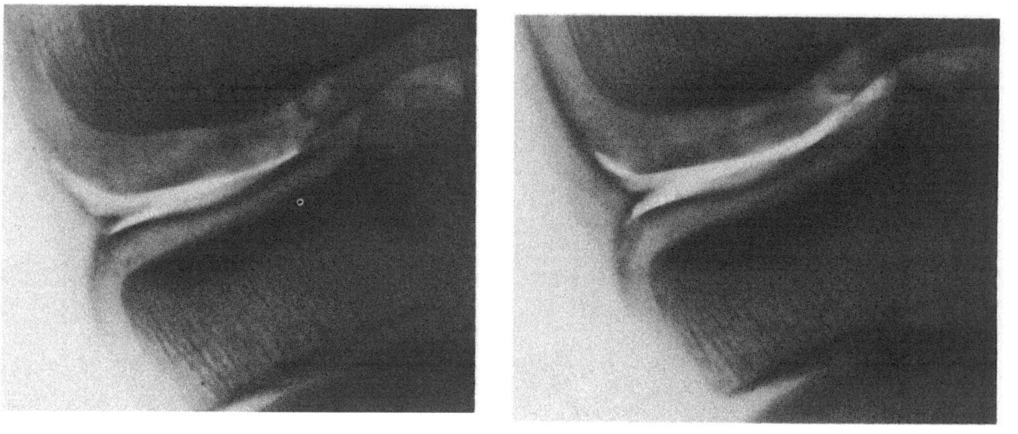

Fig. 71. Medial meniscus. Normal, sharply defined regenerate

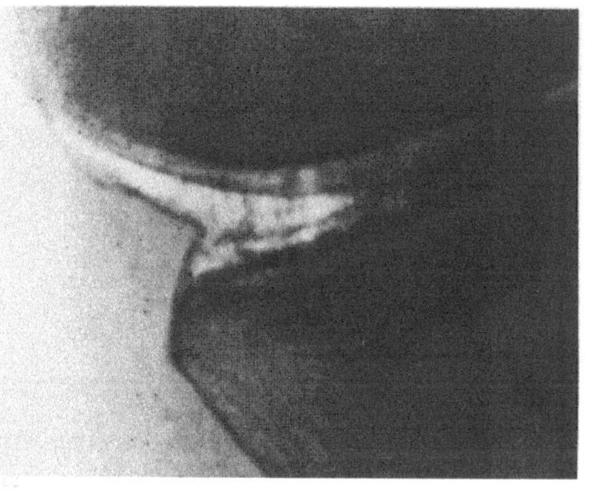

Fig. 72. Medial meniscus. Normal, sharply defined regenerate

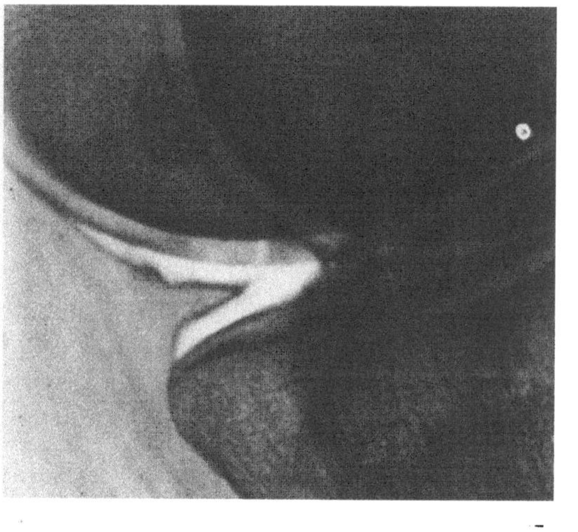

Fig. 73. Posterior horn of medial meniscus. Normal, sharply defined regenerate

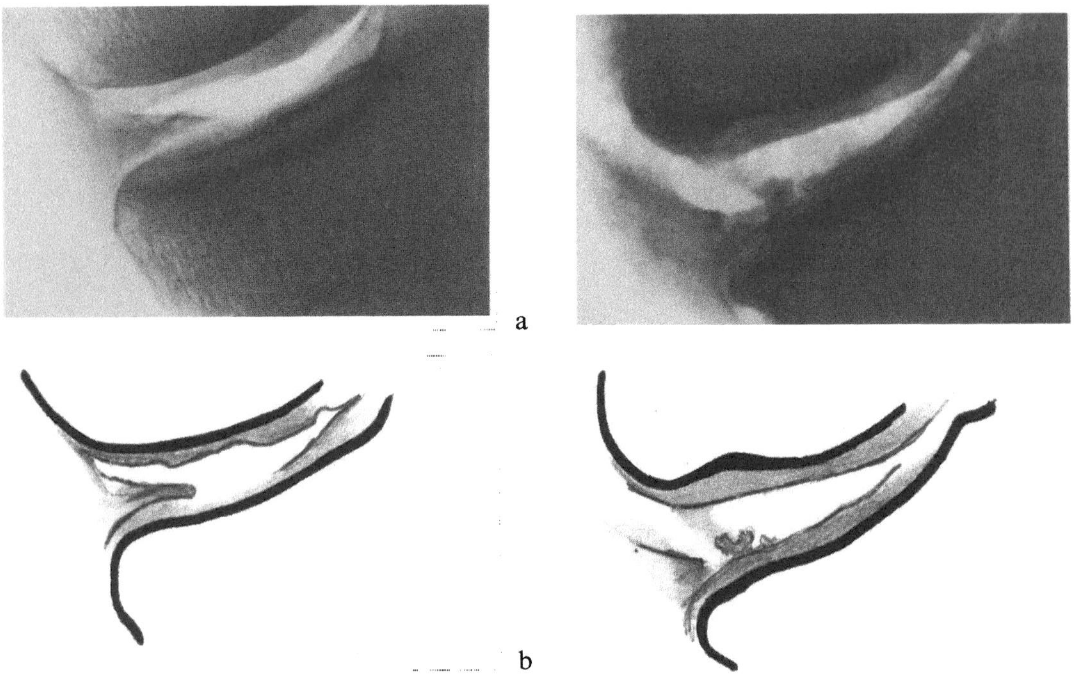

Fig. 74a and b. Partial medial meniscectomy. The two radiographs a and and b (and accessory drawings) show cartilaginous meniscal remnant and secondary degeneration of meniscal cartilage and articular cartilage

Smillie (1944) excised damaged regenerates in five patients. In all cases, marked lesions of the cruciate ligaments, collateral ligaments, and capsule were found in addition to the damaged regenerates. A meniscal remnant left in situ, without degeneration, is sometimes not readily distinguishable from a regenerate. Thiemann and Fischer (1970) demonstrated that a large percentage of patients showed degenerative lesions of meniscal fragments left in situ at operation. Such degenerative lesions are arthrographically visible as ill-defined contours of the meniscal remnant, due to imbibition of the meniscal surface with contrast medium (Figs. 74 and 75). The presence of a meniscal remnant is indicated by a meniscal width of 9 mm at the level of the anterior horn and midportion and of 15 mm at the level of the posterior horn. When these dimensions are 3–8 mm and less than 15 mm, respectively, it is impossible to differentiate between meniscal remnants and meniscal regenerates solely on the basis of measurements. The histologic differentiation between regenerate and meniscal remnant poses no problem, because a regenerate contains no cartilaginous tissue.

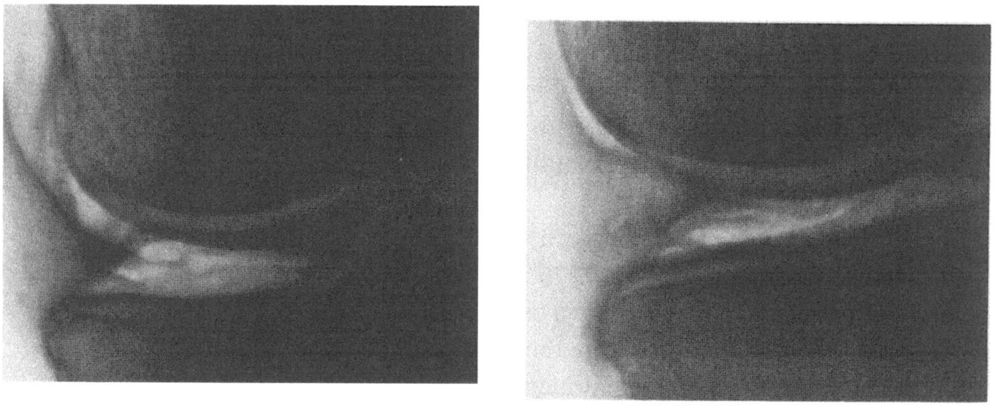

Fig. 75. Partial medial meniscectomy. Large cartilaginous meniscal remnant with secondary cartilage degeneration

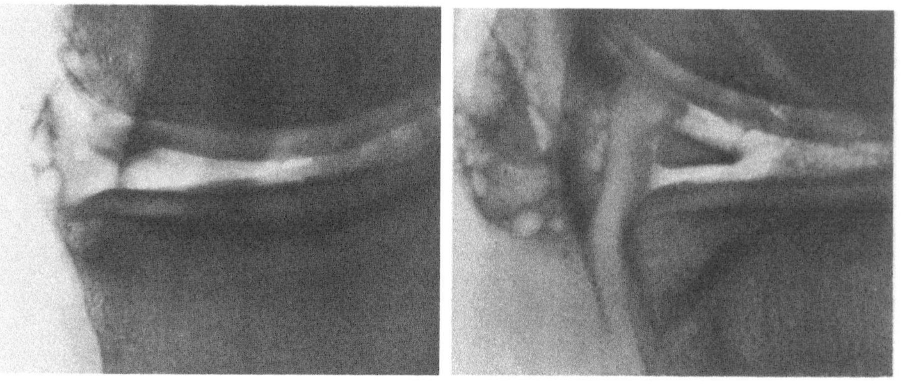

Fig. 76. After two medial meniscectomies: evidently detached remnant of posterior horn. Semimembranosogastrocnemial bursa

3.7 Correlation Between Arthrography and Arthroscopy

Arthroscopy of the knee joint, which has evolved to a very good technique in the past decade, makes it possible to diagnose a wide range of intra-articular lesions (Jackson, 1968, 1972; Eikelaar, 1975). For a detailed description of this method we refer to the pertinent literature. Arthroscopy makes it possible to examine synovium, cruciate ligaments, articular cartilage, retropatellar cartilage, and menisci. In many cases, however, it is difficult to visualize the entire medial posterior horn. When the anterior cruciate ligament is intact, the posterior cruciate ligament is likewise not readily visualized. To facilitate diagnosis of meniscal rupture, the arthroscopist often inserts a small needle at the periphery of the meniscus to establish whether part of the meniscus can be luxated (Figs. 77 and 78 see page 142). Another possibility is to take synovial biopsy specimens during arthroscopy; aimed removal of small detached meniscal fragments is also possible.

We studied the correlation between double contrast arthrography and arthroscopy in a group of 226 patients. All were first examined arthrographically, then arthroscopically.

A positive correlation between the two methods was found in 102 of 111 patients with medial meniscal lesions (92%). Arthrography yielded dubious findings in 4 patients (4%) and false positive results in 5 (4%). No false negative result was recorded.

Table 2. Correlation between double contrast arthrography and arthroscopy in 111 medial meniscal lesions

	Arthrography		Arthroscopy	
Correct +	102	92%	90	81%
Dubious	4	4%	3	3%
False +	5	4%	–	–
False –	–	–	18	16%
Total	111		111	

At arthroscopy, 90 of the 111 medial meniscal lesions were correctly diagnosed (81%), the result being dubious in 3 patients (3%). The arthroscopic result was false negative in 18 patients (16%). The data are presented in Table 2. The medial meniscal

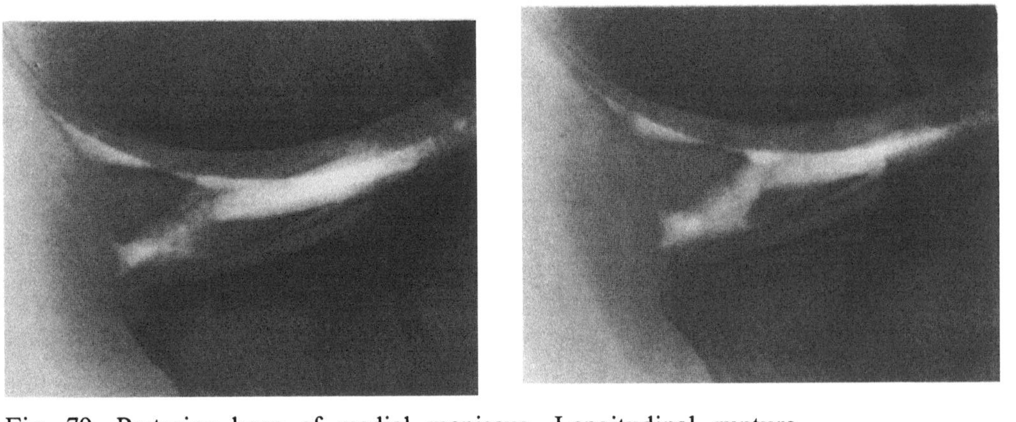

Fig. 79. Posterior horn of medial meniscus. Longitudinal rupture type IIa. No arthroscopic lesion! Conclusion: false negative arthroscopic result

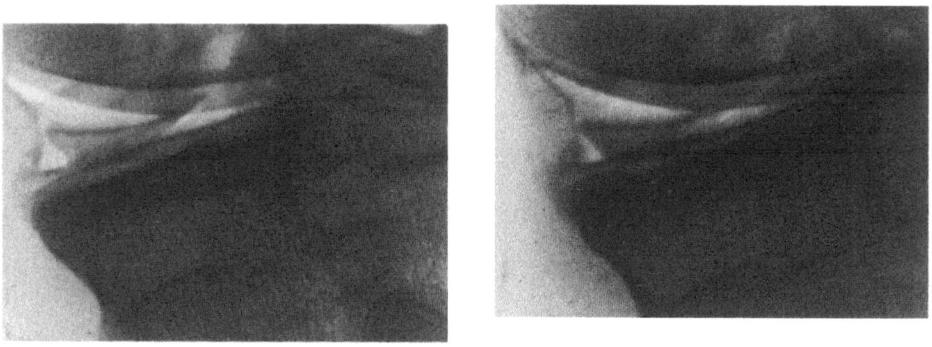

Fig. 80. Posterior horn of medial meniscus. Longitudinal rupture type IIa. No arthroscopic lesion! Conclusion: false negative arthroscopic result

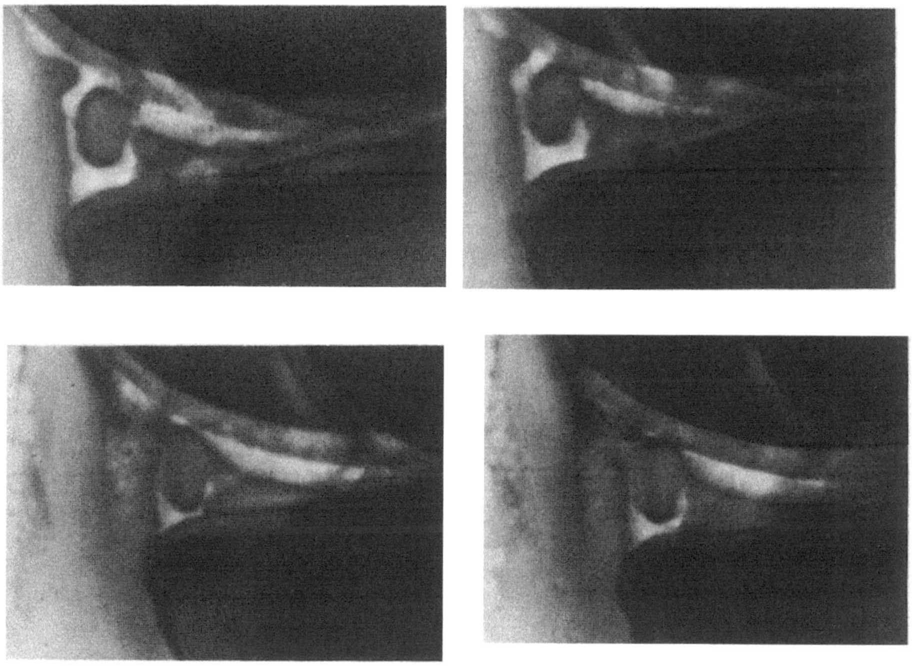

Fig. 81. Posterior horn of medial meniscus. Two longitudinal ruptures of the meniscus. No arthroscopic lesion! Conclusion: false negative arthroscopic result

ruptures not identified by arthroscopy were nearly all localized in the medial posterior horn. Evaluation of this area poses problems for the arthroscopist. The central margin of the meniscus can usually be evaluated without difficulty. Examination of the upper surface of the meniscus is not so easy. If the central margin of the meniscus is sharply depicted and needle manipulation fails to luxate the ruptured meniscal fragment, then the arthroscopist is unable to diagnose medial meniscal rupture. The diagnosis on the basis of intra-articular changes is therefore not comprehensive if the examination is restricted to arthroscopy.

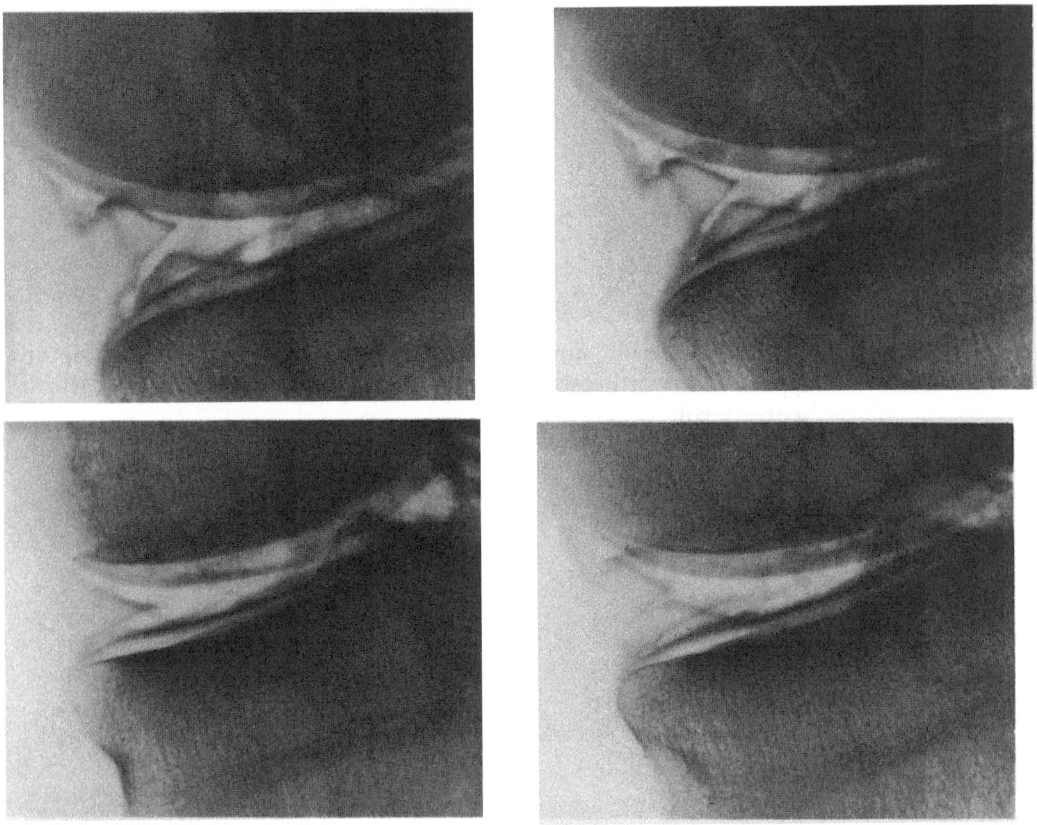

Fig. 82. Posterior horn of medial meniscus. Evident oblique longitudinal rupture of the meniscus. No arthroscopic lesion! Conclusion: false negative arthroscopic result

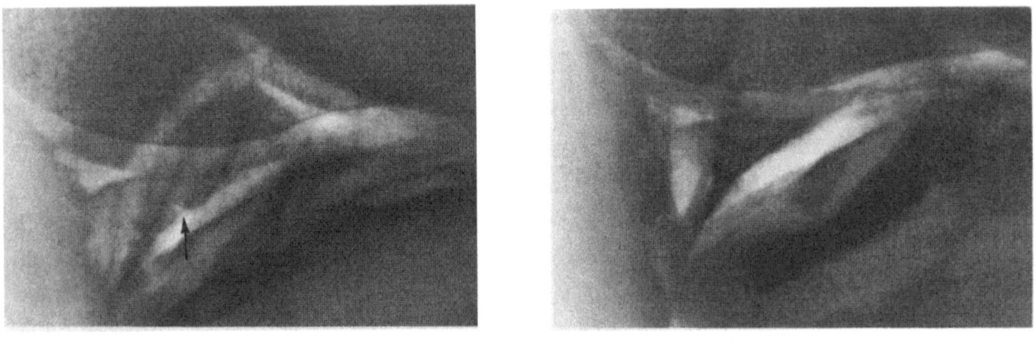

Fig. 83. Posterior horn of lateral meniscus. Tangential rupture on the underside of the meniscus (*arrow*). No arthroscopic lesion

This examination should be preceded by arthrography. The two methods are supplemental and each has its diagnostic value (Figs. 79–82; also Figs. 40, 42, and 43).

In the examination of 67 lateral meniscal lesions the accuracy of arthrography was 90%, with false positive results in 2 cases (3%) and false negative results in 5 (7%). Arthroscopy of the lateral meniscus proved to be substantially more accurate than that of the medial meniscus. Of 67 lateral meniscal lesions, 66 were correctly diagnosed (98%), in only one patient (2%) was a false negative arthroscopic result recorded. This patient had a small tangential incisure of the lateral posterior horn, which was arthroscopically overlooked (Fig. 83, Table 3).

Table 3. Correlation between double contrast arthrography and arthroscopy in 67 lateral meniscal lesions

	Arthrography		Arthroscopy	
Correct +	60	90%	66	98%
Dubious	–	–	–	–
False +	2	3%	–	–
False –	5	7%	1	2%
Total	67		67	

In the entire group of 178 medial and lateral meniscal lesions the accuracy of arthrography proved to be 91,5% and that of arthroscopy was 88% (Table 4). The false positive results in examination of the medial meniscus were caused by synovial hypertrophy and a ruptured anterior cruciate ligament in one patient (Fig. 137). In the five cases in which arthrography of the lateral meniscus gave a false negative result, subsequent arthroscopy revealed three longitudinal and two transverse ruptures of the meniscus.

The above study gives an impression of the correlation between double contrast arthrography and arthroscopy. In the literature, the reliability of arthrography in the diagnosis of meniscal lesions is indicated by many authors as 90%–100% (Wiener, 1967; Thijn, 1968; Kiss and Moir, 1968; Jelaso and Usar, 1968; Butt, 1969; Nicholas et al., 1970; Freiberger et al., 1966; Lindblom, 1948; Savastano, 1974; McBeath et al., 1972; Romaniuk and Thomas, 1968). Given a minor lesion in the arthrogram or a dubious arthrographic diagnosis, subsequent arthroscopy is often performed instead of an operation. Consequently, the accuracy

Table 4. Correlation between double contrast arthrography and arthroscopy in 226 patients. The table indicates the correlation for the medial, the lateral, and the total number of meniscal lesions

	Arthrography				Arthroscopy			Number of lesions
	Correct	Dubious	False+	False−	Correct	Dubious	False−	
Medial meniscus	92%	4%	4%	–	81%	3%	16%	111
Lateral meniscus	90%	–	3%	7%	98%	–	2%	67
Medial and lateral meniscus	91,5%	2%	4%	2,5%	88%	1%	11%	178

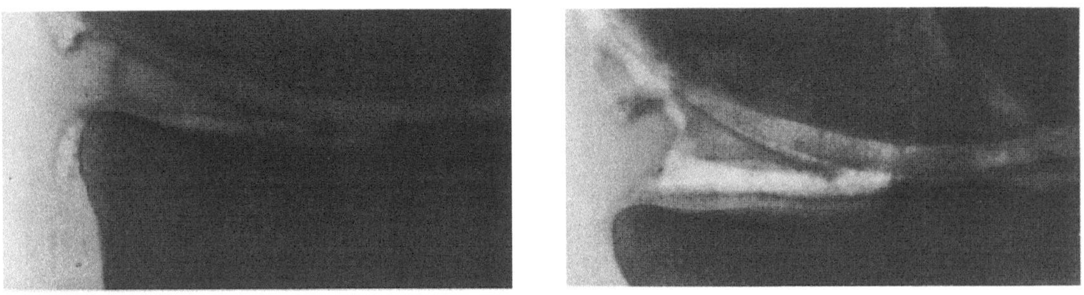

Fig. 84. Medial meniscus. These projections demonstrate the importance of adequate dilatation of the articular cavity examined, facilitating diagnosis of a longitudinal rupture

rates reported in the literature on the correlation between arthrography and operation are likely to be optimistic and would have been considerably lower if arthroscopy had been carried out in all cases. In the past decade we observed a decrease in rate of accuracy from 93% (Thijn, 1968) to 91,5%, despite increased technical sophistication. The former rate was calculated on the basis of the correlation between arthrography and operation, whereas in the latter the correlation between arthrography and arthroscopy was considered.

4 Lesions of the Patellofemoral Joint

4.1 Anatomy and Physiology of the Patellofemoral Joint

The two femoral condyles are dorsally separated by a deep groove not lined with cartilage: the intercondylar fossa, which ventrally continues into the trochlear sulcus. The latter is lined with cartilage and constitutes part of the patellar surface of the femur. Although shallow, this groove is nevertheless a well-defined boundary between the medial and the lateral femoral condyle.

Comparative anatomic studies have revealed an unmistakable relation between the ability to extend the knee completely and the depth of the trochlear sulcus. In anthropoids, which cannot fully extend the knee, the patellar surface of the femur is virtually flat. Even in man, the above described sulcus is not completely developed until after age 12. In human adults, the sulcus is not always equally deep, and the lateral femoral condyle is not always equally prominent. An aberrant form is often found in patients suffering from habitual luxation of the patella. This will later be discussed in detail.

The femoral condyles are lined with cartilage of varying thickness. In the central area of the patellar femoral surface the layer of cartilage is about 3–4 mm thick, becoming thinner toward the periphery.

The patella is a flat, triangular piece of bone, with the apex on the distal side. With the exception of the posterior surface, virtually the entire surface is attached to the extensor apparatus. The anterior aspect of the patella is slightly convex, with sagittal grooves and four or five nutrient foramina. The posterior aspect of the patella is covered by a layer of hyaline cartilage which accounts for a quarter of the total thickness of the patella. This 4–5 mm layer is the thickest layer of cartilage found in human joints. The surface bulges and can be divided into a lateral and a medial articular surface, separated by a ridge called the linea eminens. In cross section, the patella shows a triangular shape so that it fits snugly into the trochlear sulcus of the femur.

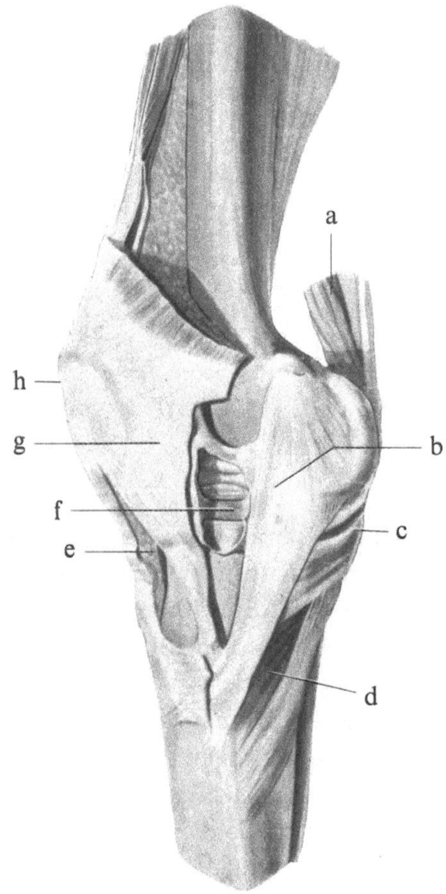

Fig. 85. Medial view of the knee joint (after W. Spalteholz, 1954)
a. M. semimembranosus
b. Ligamentum collaterale mediale
c. Tendo musculi semimembranosi
d. Musculus popliteus
e. Corpus adiposum genus
f. Meniscus medialis
g. Retinaculum patellae mediale
h. Patella

The articular surfaces of the patella are usually concave, and as a rule the lateral surface is distinctly larger than the medial. With the knee fully extended, only the caudal facets are in contact with the patellar surface of the femur; with the knee in extreme extension, only the two cranial facets are in contact with the condyles.

With the knee extended and the quadriceps femoris muscle taut, at best only the caudal part of the patella is still in contact with the most proximal portion of the cartilage-lined patellar surface of the femur. Most of the patella rests against the anterior aspect of the femur, which at this level is covered only by the synovial membrane of the suprapatellar recess. In that case the patellar apex on the anterior side lies 2–3 cm above the tibial plateau.

With the knee extended and the quadriceps femoris muscle relaxed, the patella sags distally. Its apex then lies at the level of the tibial plateau. In this situation the patella can be passively moved up and down in caudocranial, as well as in mediolateral

Fig. 86. Anterior view of the knee joint (after W. Spalteholz, 1954)
a. Bursa suprapatellaris
b. Ligamentum cruciatum posterius
c. Condylus medialis femoris
d. Ligamentum cruciatum anterius
e. Meniscus medialis
f. Plicae alares
g. Facies articularis patellae
h. Bursa suprapatellaris
i. Meniscus lateralis
j. Plica synovialis infrapatellaris
k. Condylus lateralis femoris

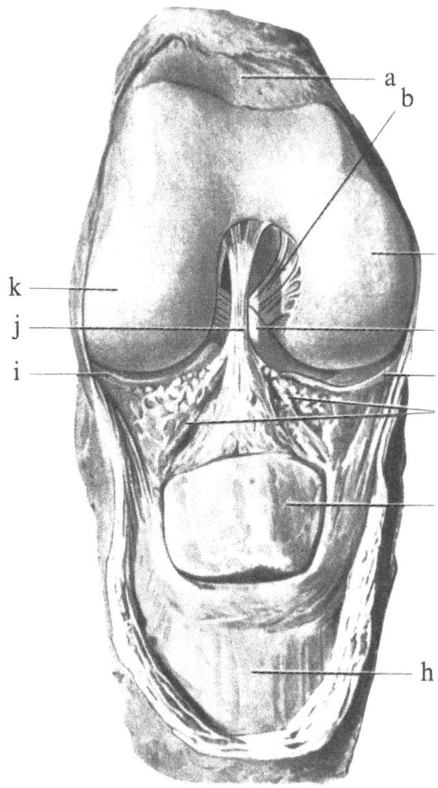

direction. In some cases this mobility is greatly increased, e.g., in patients with habitual luxation of the patella.

The capsule on the anterior side of the knee consists of the fibrous membrane, which for the most part is made up of the aponeurosis of the quadriceps femoris muscle and the synovial membrane. Both constitute part of the capsule of the knee joint (Chap. 6).

The quadriceps femoris muscle has four component parts: the rectus femoris, the vastus medialis, the vastus lateralis, and the vastus intermedius muscle. Distally, these largely converge in the broad aponeurosis of the quadriceps tendon, which partly inserts on the superior aspect of the patella (Fig. 85). Some of the fibers extend past the ventral aspect of the patella to the patellar ligament. This ligament has a length of about 5–6 cm and a width of 2–3 cm; it is about 0.5 cm thick and extends from the apex of the patella to the tibial tuberosity. Medial and lateral fibers of the quadriceps femoris muscle form the patellar retinaculum. This retinaculum is part of the extensor apparatus of the knee

and, upon contraction of the quadriceps femoris muscle, forms a firm aponeurosis which fixes the patella in lateral direction as well. Beneath this superficial layer of longitudinal fibers, the transverse fibers of the transverse patellar retinaculum extend. They connect the patella to the medial as well as to the lateral femoral epicondyle. Laterally, these fibers are reinforced by the fibers of the iliotibial tract, which extends in the same direction. Thus fixation of the patella in four directions is ensured: on the superior side by the quadriceps tendon, on the inferior side by the patellar ligament, and laterally as well as medially by the longitudinal fibers of the retinaculum. The transverse patellar retinacula, which connect the patella to the femoral epicondyles, are likewise important for fixation.
Between the synovial membrane and the fibrous membrane, a thin layer of adipose tissue is present proximal to the patella. Distal to the patella, i.e., beneath the patellar ligament, a larger amount of adipose tissue is present: the adipose body of the knee, also known as Hoffa body. This adipose body forms folds protruding into the articular cavity: the alar folds. From this site, a synovial fold extends in the sagittal plane to the anterior part of the intercondylar fossa; this is the infrapatellar synovial fold (mucous ligament), which can locally divide the articular cavity into two parts (Figs. 86 and 132).

4.2 Articular Cartilage

4.2.1 Histology

The cartilage consists of cartilage cells, chondrocytes embedded in the mucoid intercellular substance in which collagenous fibers extend virtually parallel to the cartilage surface in the more superficial layers, and virtually perpendicular to the cartilage surface in the deeper layers. The tensile strength of the cartilage depends on the course of these collagenous fibers. The material between the collagenous fibers is made up of mucopolysaccharides and glycoproteins. The total amount of mucopolysaccharides varies markedly, and the distribution over the various layers of the cartilage is not even. For example, the mucopolysaccharide content is less in the superficial than in the deeper and pericellular parts (Bollet et al., 1966; Collins et al., 1960). Water accounts for 75%–78% of the weight of patellar cartilage, which in this way corresponds with the cartilage of other joints (Linn et al., 1965). The superficial layers have the highest water concentration (Muir, 1970).

4.2.2 Nutrition of Cartilage

Since the cartilage is not vascularized, the question arises how nutrients can reach the cartilage cells. They might come from the synovia, from the subchondral bone, or from both. Trueta and Harrison (1953) found capillary vessels which, via narrow canaliculi in the subchondral bone, reached the deeper layers of the calcified cartilage. However, these deeper layers were never passed and, in view of the marked calcification, should probably be regarded as a barrier. Although nutrition of cartilage via the subchondral bone cannot be excluded with certainty, at least in adult animals this nutrition seems largely to take place via the synovial fluid. This is further corroborated by the observation that cartilage continues to live after contact with the subchondral bone is abolished. Moreover, a dye injected into the articular cavity proves to reach all layers of the cartilage (Hodge et al., 1969; Honner et al., 1971). Nutrients can enter the cartilage by simple diffusion or by active transport. Diffusion would seem to be sufficient only for the superficial layers of cartilage (Bywaters, 1937; Maroudas, 1968b). The observation that varying stress on the cartilage led to expulsion and re-uptake of fluid seemed to suggest a pump mechanism (Müller, 1929; Salter et al., 1965; Sood, 1971). This theory was supported by the observation that immobilization (i.e., discontinuation of the varying stress) led to cartilage degeneration, whereas active exercise led to swelling of cartilage and an increase in the total amount of fluid (Ekholm, 1955; Maroudas, 1968b).

4.2.3 Properties of Cartilage

The elastic properties of articular cartilage were studied in stress experiments. When the cartilage was compressed by constant stress, a time-linked deformation occurred with expulsion of water (Sokoloff, 1966; Linn et al., 1965).

The elastic properties can be explained as follows. The network of collagenous fibers extends through the calcified zone, thus connecting the cartilage to the subchondral bone. Although the exact relation between this network and the intercellular substance has remained obscure, it is assumed that the collagenous fibers mechanically immobilize the glycoproteins (Benninghof, 1925; Freemann, 1973). In view of the osmotic values of the filling material, water is attracted, so that pressure is exerted. In response to a mechanical influence the water can be expulsed, but this requires some time (Harkness, 1968; MacCutchen, 1965). When a large surface is subjected to stress (e.g., in the hip joint), it takes long before the visible amount of water is expulsed (Paul, 1965). When the stress is only briefly applied, hardly any water is expulsed, and the reaction of the cartilage is based on the elasticity, which causes only deformation not a decrease in volume. Equilibrium after protracted stress, with expulsion of water, is based on resumption of osmotic equilibrium on a lower level due to a relatively higher concentration of glycoproteins (Linn et al., 1965). Continuous marked stress causes expulsion of a large amount of water, and marked deformation. During dynamic and especially during brief stress, marked forces arise within the collagenous structure. Perhaps a fatigue rupture of the fibers can occur on this basis. Deficiency of glycoproteins would exert an unfavorable influence on this.

4.2.4 Cartilage Degeneration

When the surface of slightly damaged cartilage is colored with india ink and microscopically examined, superficial fissures are observed which often are parallel, but sometimes show a serrated or more irregular pattern. Examination of histologic specimens shows that the fissures are parallel to the collagenous fibers. In the case of fissures which extend slightly into the surface of the cartilage, the course is likewise parallel to the collagenous fibers, and small, initially still attached flakes develop (Fig. 87 see page 142). A more severe lesion involves the deeper layers as well, and the division is then more perpendicular to the cartilage surface (Collins, 1949; Meachim et al., 1965).
At palpation, a soft consistency of the cartilage is the first change found in chondropathy. Some investigators regard this changed consistency (believed to be based on a decreased amount of mucopolysaccharides) as the change on the basis of which the fissures develop. The decrease in mucopolysaccharides, they maintain, is still reversible (Ficat, 1970a, 1973). Freeman (1973), however, maintains that the decrease in mucopolysaccharides

results from leakage due to rupture of the collagenous fibers. Progression of the changes gradually leads to the formation of deep fissures and crumbling of the cartilage, until finally the subchondral bone is exposed.

In his thesis Rijnks (1976) distinguished four grades of cartilage degeneration (chondropathy) of the patella:

Grade I: The cartilage shows superficial fissures which initially are only microscopically demonstrable. The amount of mucopolysaccharides is decreased, and the amount of water increased (which of the two changes occurs first is obscure). The cartilaginous changes are manifested by a softening and slight swelling of the focus in relation to the unaffected tissue and a light-yellow discoloration.

Grade II: The fissures extend in depth and become macroscopically visible.

Grade III: The fissures become deeper and locally extend as far as the subchondral bone. Flakes of cartilage detach themselves from the surface.

Grade IV: Ulceration occurs, with local total destruction of cartilage. At the periphery of the lesions there is often a gradual transition to healthy cartilage, with the various grades of degeneration (already mentioned) occurring side by side.

4.2.5 Normal Radiologic Anatomy

Although computerized axial tomography (CT) is of great importance in the diagnosis of lesions elsewhere in the body, it seems to have little value in examining the knee joint and the patellofemoral joint. With CT, cross sections of the patellofemoral joint can be visualized without injection of contrast medium, and these are more or less comparable to tangential projections of this joint (Fig. 88).

The relations between the bone fragments in the patellofemoral joint can be evaluated in a simple manner on the basis of lateral and tangential radiographs. The technique has been described in Chap. 2. The relation between patella and femoral condyles is best observed in the tangential projections (Fig. 89). Instead of these projections, many investigators prefer to examine the patients in prone position with the knee in extreme flexion, aiming the central beam tangentially at the knee joint. This projection can give rise to the impression that the distance between one of the posterior facets of the patella and the femoral condyle is reduced. The tangential projection with the patient sitting,

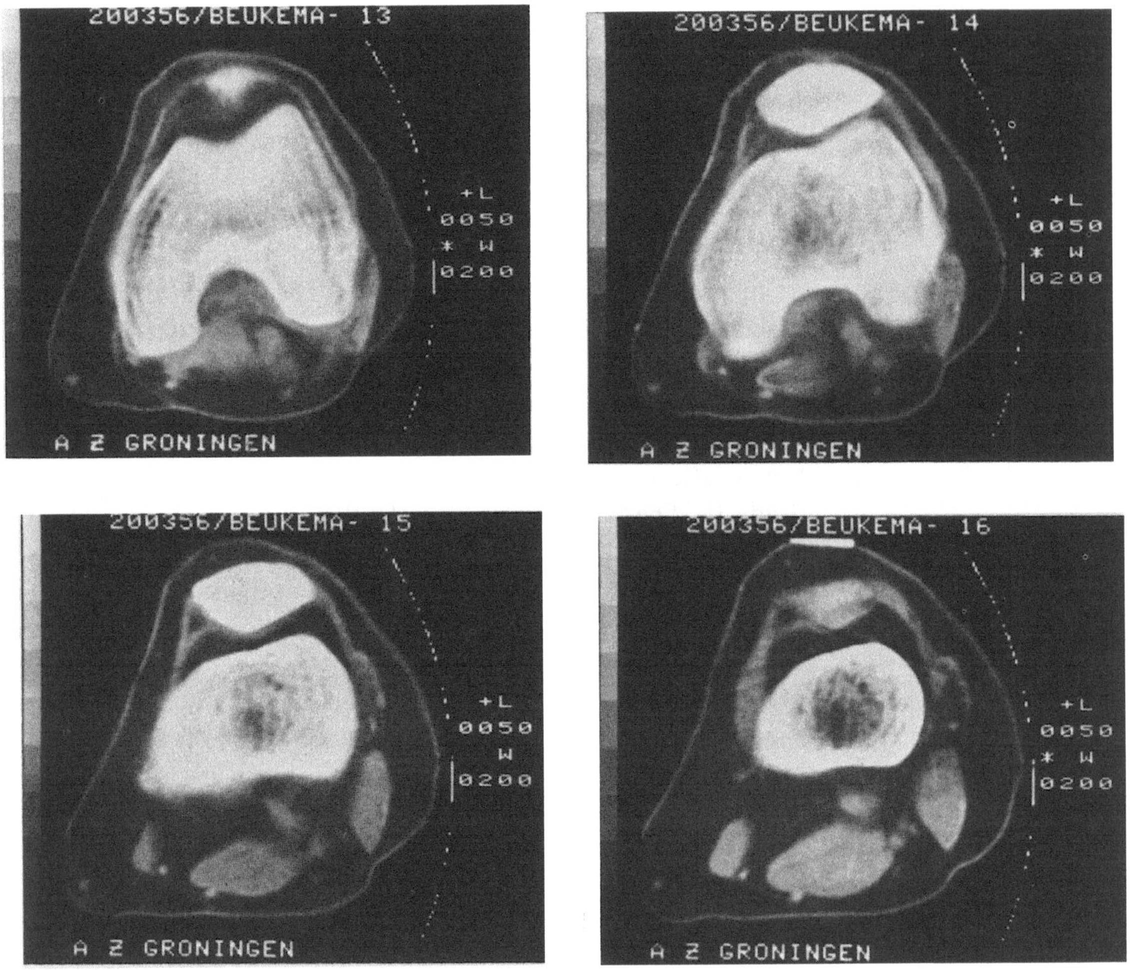

Fig. 88. Computerized tomography (CT) of the knee joint. The relation between patella and femoral condyles and the joint capsule, and the soft tissues, are clearly visible. However, an exact assessment of the patellofemoral joint is not possible

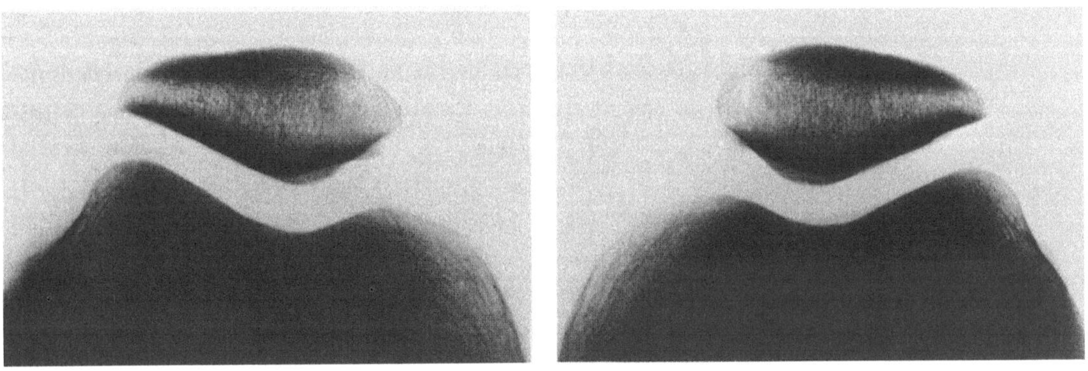

Fig. 89. Tangential projection of the patella. The relation between patella and femoral condyles can be adequately assessed

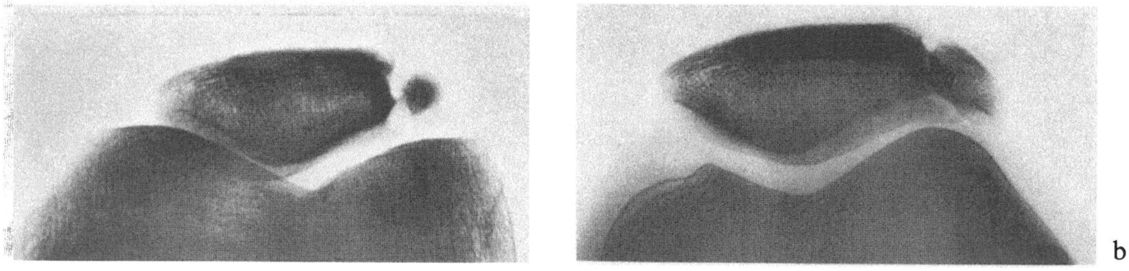

a b

Fig. 90 a and b. Patella bipartita. (a) Projection with the patient prone and the knee in maximal flexion. (b) Tangential projection with the patient sitting. In this way the relation between patella and femoral condyles is best visualized. The narrowing of the medial intra-articular space visible in (a) proves to be spurious

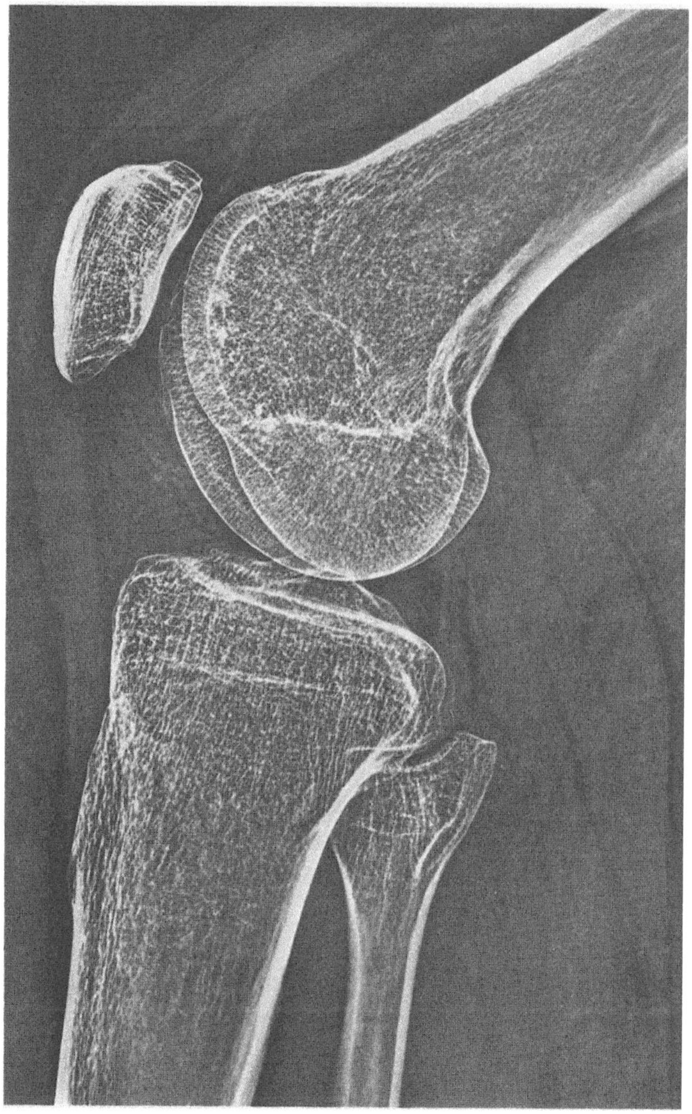

Fig. 91. Xerography. Adequate depiction of the soft tissues around the knee joint

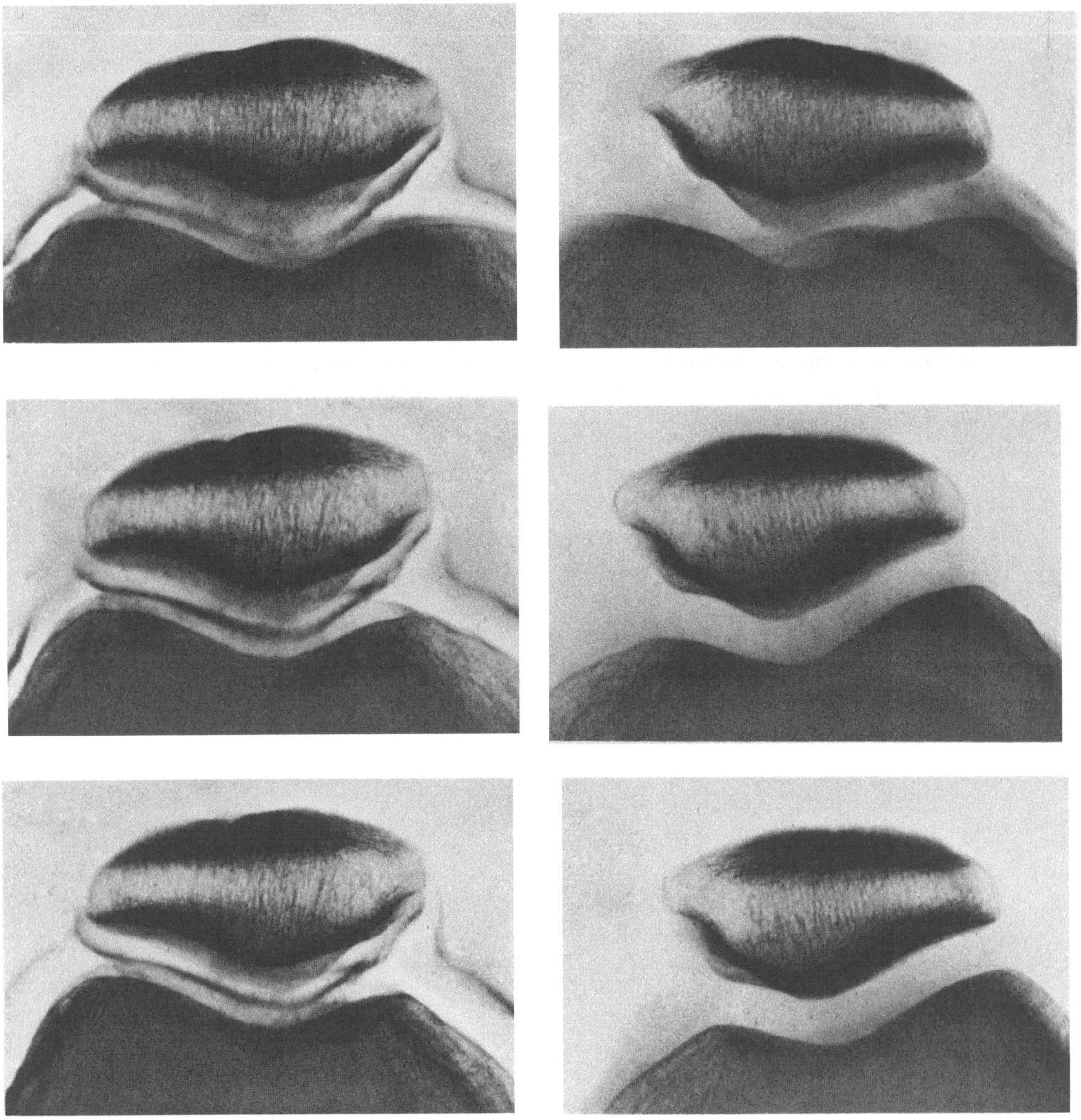

Fig. 92. Tangential projections of the patella with the knee joint in 30°, 60°, and 90° flexion

however, gives a more accurate depiction of the relations (Fig. 90).

The soft tissues around the patella are best visualized in soft-tissue projections made with low kilovoltage or in xerograms (Fig. 91). The cartilage of the patella and femoral condyles is best visualized by double contrast arthrography, making three tangential projections with the knee flexed 30°, 60°, and 90°, respectively (Fig. 92), so that each of the projections depicts different facets of the retropatellar surface. In addition to these serial tangential projections, lateral detail projections are used (Chap. 2; Figs. 7, 93 and 94).

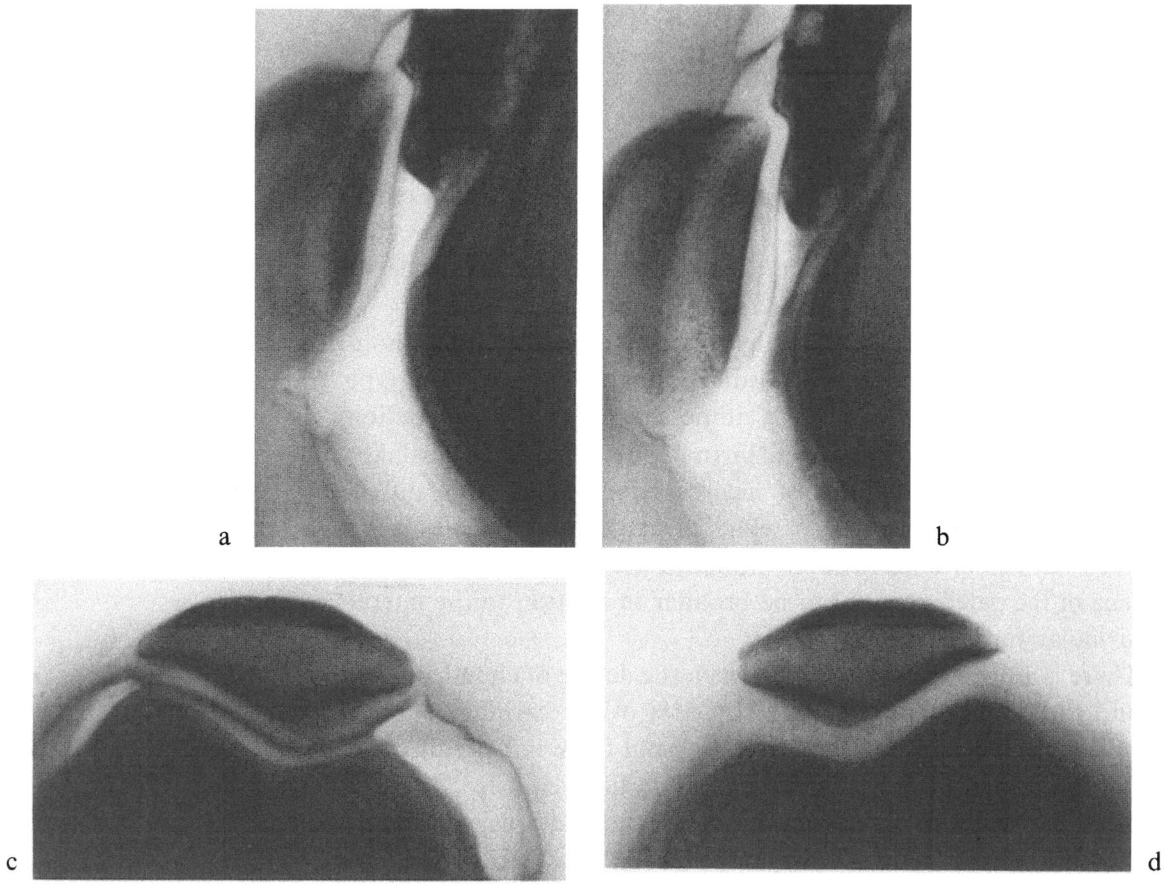

Fig. 93a–d. Lateral (a and b) and tangential (c) projection of the patellofemoral joint in the same knee. Sharp demarcation of the normal retropatellar cartilage. Tangential projection of the other knee joint (d)

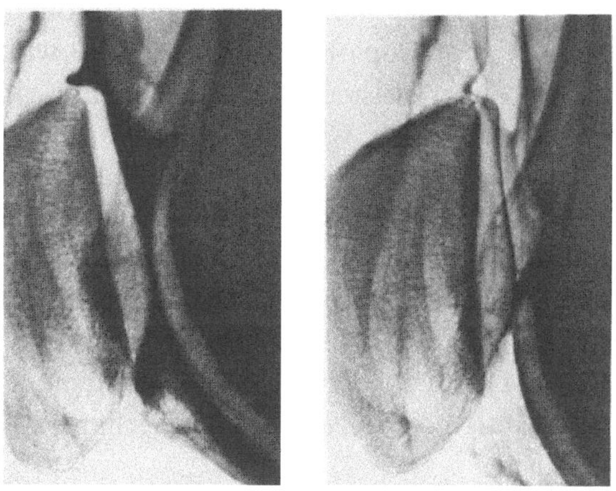

Fig. 94. Lateral projections of the patellofemoral joint. The articular surface at single contrast and at double contrast arthrography

4.3 Etiology of Patellar Chondropathy

4.3.1 General Aspects

In a postmortem study of 79 patellae, Rijnks (1976) found patellar chondropathy in 68% of cases. These lesions were especially frequent in patients of more advanced age. The incidence of chondropathy was 86% in the age group over 50 and 28% in the age group under 30. The high incidences indicate that chondropathy probably does not produce severe symptoms. The type of cartilage lesion may be of importance for the production of symptoms. Deep fissures and virtually detached cartilage flakes can give rise to symptoms of incarceration. Apart from differences in dimensions, the patellae of males and females were not found to differ. However, in males the medial articular surface of the patella proved to be broader in relation to the lateral articular surface of the female.

There is a significant relation between the degree of chondropathy and the extent of the lesions. All parts of the cartilage surface of the patella can show chondropathy, but there is a predilection for the medial facet and the area of the linea eminens. In 77% of all patellae with chondropathy, the severest lesions were localized medially or centrally, while the lateral articular surface was much less frequently involved (in only 14% of cases were the severest lesions localized here).

Rijnks' study also showed that 44 of the 196 arthroscopically examined patients (22%) already had a chondropathy at the first operation for a meniscal lesion. Of the 16 patients who underwent a second meniscectomy, 5 (about 30%) showed chondropathy. Patellar chondropathy was likewise found in 17 out of 24 meniscectomy patients (71%) whose persistent symptoms led to arthroscopy. In the latter group of patients there was nearly always chondropathy of the tibiofemoral joint.

Patellar chondropathy can cause pain, which is often localized on the anterior side of the knee and can be aggravated by protracted sitting with the knee flexed, ascending stairs, and squatting. At palpation of the patella the patient often indicates pain around it. However, pain which occurs during motion of the patella on the underlying structure is the clearest indication of patellar chondropathy. Demonstration of crepitation during the examination is of diagnostic importance.

Rijnks (1976) divided the etiological factors in patellar chondropathy into mechanical and non-mechanical lesions of the patellar cartilage.

4.3.2 Mechanical Lesions of the Patellar Cartilage

The group of mechanical lesions of the patellar cartilage encompasses exogenous causes such as: direct lesion of the patella, overstress, and lesion of the cartilage resulting from fracture consolidation in an abnormal position. An abnormal structure of the patellofemoral joint constitutes an endogenous mechanical factor.

4.3.2.1 Exogenous Factors

Direct Lesion of the Patella (Fig. 95). In the older literature, direct lesion of the patella was regarded as the sole cause of patellar chondropathy. In this context Büdinger (1906, 1908) already mentioned the aspect of cartilage lesions. The fissures were reminiscent of cartilage fractures as a result of an injury. Since many patients were unable to recall a definite injury, it was assumed that several minor lesions, forgotten by the patient, can also give rise to patellar chondropathy.
Bandi (1972, 1973) maintained that a healed patellar fracture, a cartilage fracture, and contusion of cartilage can lead to patellar chondropathy. In his opinion femoral and tibial fractures consolidated in an abnormal position, hemarthros, hydrops, immobilization in a plaster cast and dystrophy are also possible etiological factors.
In his patients with unilateral symptoms based on patellar chondropathy, Rijnks (1976) often found indications of past injuries of precisely these knee joints. It therefore seems likely that a traumatic etiology is often involved in unilateral knee symptoms,

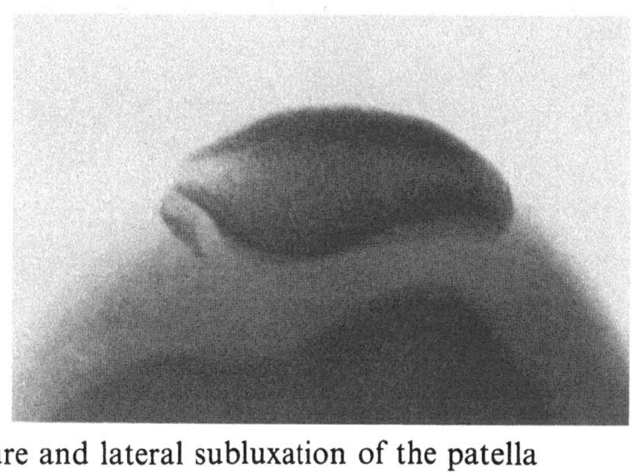

Fig. 95. Patellar fracture and lateral subluxation of the patella

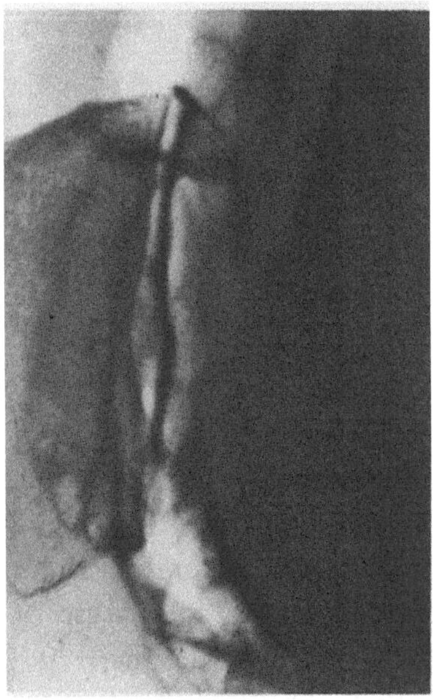

Fig. 96. Female, age 17. Fracture of the femur and lower leg at age 12. At present, marked retropatellar chondropathy. Retropatellar cartilage severely reduced

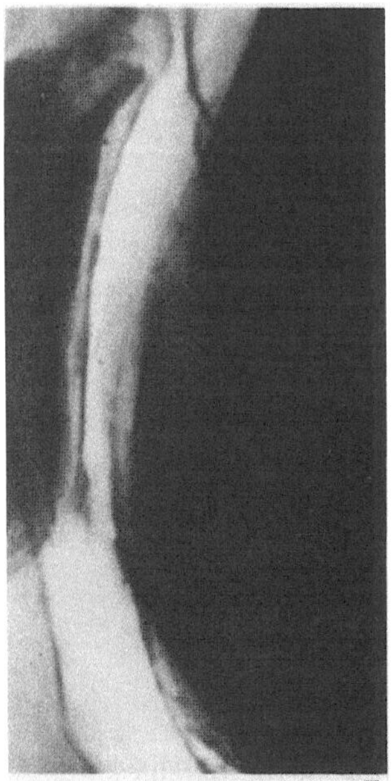

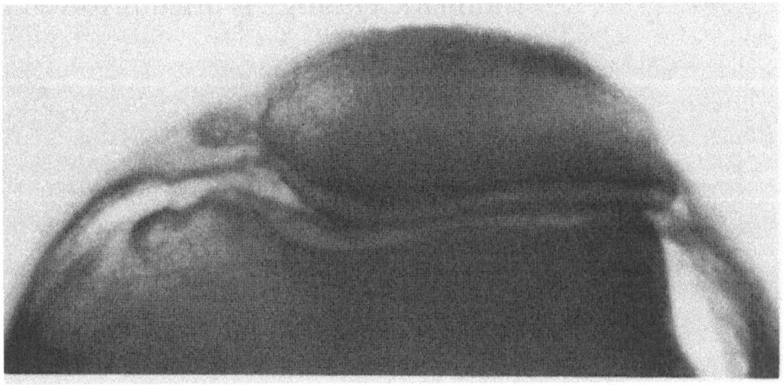

Fig. 97. Female, age 19. Situation after quadriceps transplantation. Marked patellar chondropathy

whereas bilateral symptoms are more often associated with an abnormal structure of the patellofemoral joint.

Overstress. It seems likely that overstress on the patellofemoral joint exerts an influence on the development of a chondropathy and its symptoms (Bandi, 1974; Outerbridge, 1961), although Rijnks (1976) found no indications to this effect.

Fractures. Rotation abnormalities remaining after femoral fracture can lead to overstress on the patellofemoral joint (Van Duyn, 1977). Rotation errors at reposition give rise to changes of pressure in the patellofemoral joint. Together with possible traumatic factors, these can readily explain chondropathy of the patellofemoral joint (Fig. 96). This category also includes retropatellar chondropathy, which can result from transplanting the quadriceps tendon – an operation performed in the case of habitual luxation of the patella (Fig. 97).

4.3.2.2 Endogenous Factors

Abnormal development (dysplasia) of the patellofemoral joint can place the cartilage under considerable stress, thus giving rise to patellar chondropathy. The dysplasia as a rule involves all the structures of the patellofemoral joint: musculature, capsule, patella, and femoral condyles.

Patellar Dysplasia. Given adequate contact between the articular surfaces of the patella and the femoral condyles, the weight is distributed over the largest possible surface area. A detailed study of the contact between these articular surfaces was made by Wiberg (1941) who, on the basis of tangential radiographs, distinguished three types of patella (Fig. 98).
Type I: The medial and the lateral articular surface are of equal size and concave shape.
Type II: The medial articular surface is of concave shape but unmistakably smaller than the lateral articular surface.
Type III: The medial articular surface is even smaller (less than half the size of the lateral surface) and of convex shape.
Wiberg's type III corresponds with type II/III described by Baumgartl (1964) but shows a flat medial articular surface. Baumgartl's type IV shows a medial articular surface with a concave and a convex part (Fig. 98). In addition Ficat (1970a, 1973) described yet another type of patella (*en béret de chasseur*), without medial articular surface (Figs. 99 and 100).

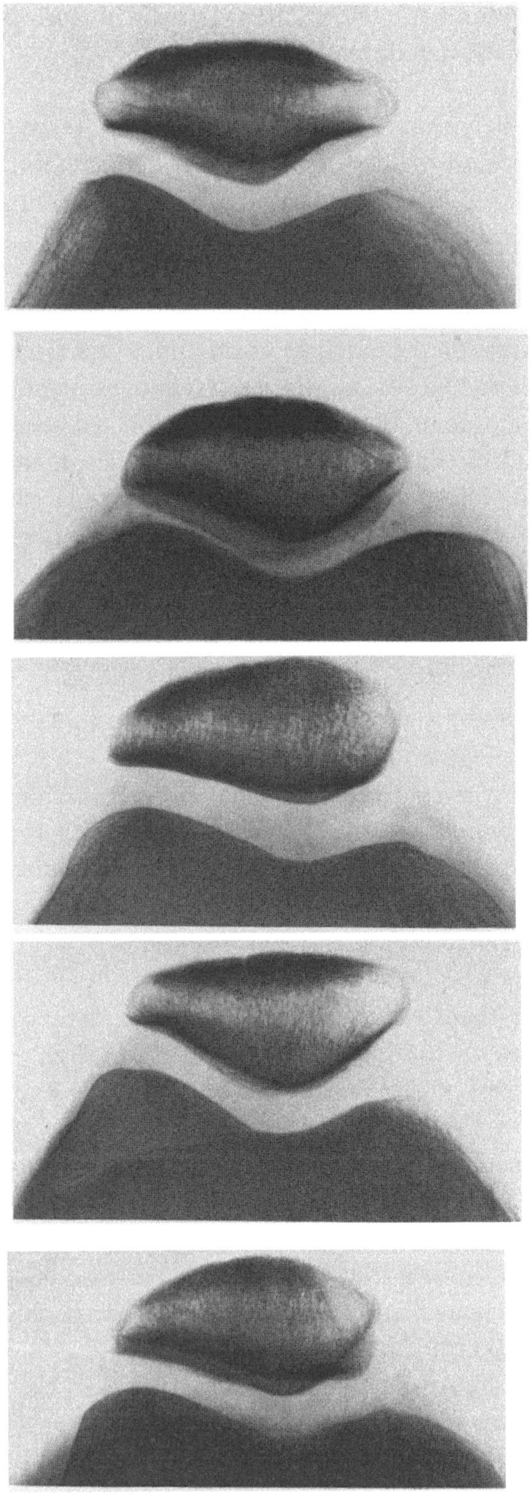

Fig. 98a–e. Patella types

a. Wiberg type I: medial and lateral facets of the patella are of equal size and concave shape

b. Wiberg type II: the medial facet is slightly concave but smaller than the lateral facet

c. Wiberg type III: the medial facet is even smaller, and convex

d. Baumgartl type II/III: corresponds with Wiberg type III but has a flat medial facet

e. Baumgartl type IV: the medial facet has both a concave and a convex part

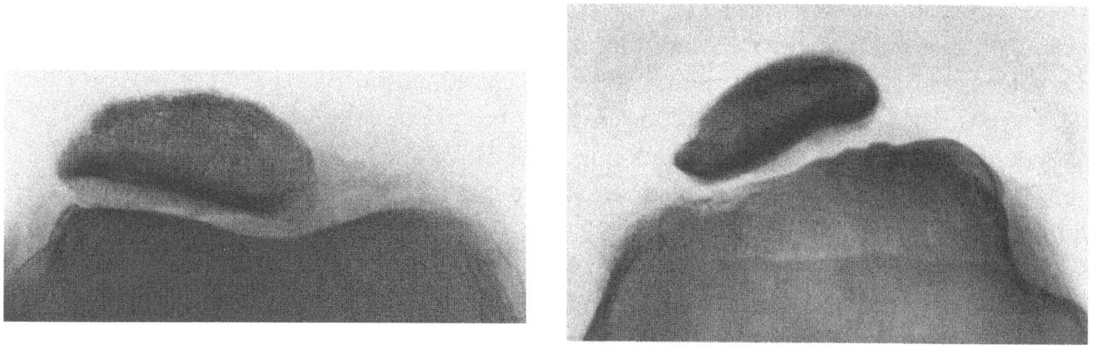

Fig. 99. Patella type "en béret de chasseur." This type is characterized by absence of the medial facet

a 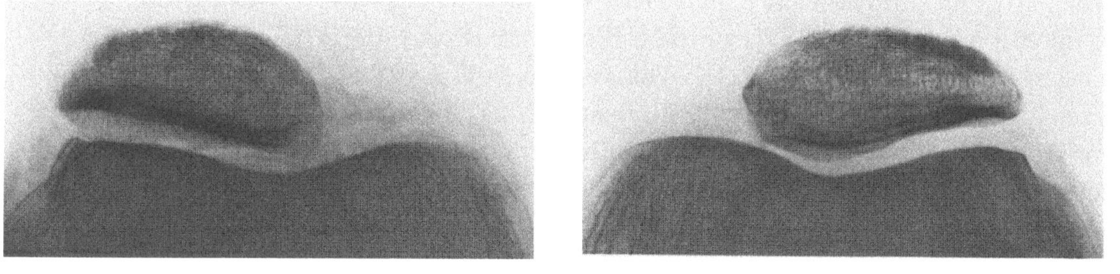 b

Fig. 100a and b. Patellar dysplasia. (a) Patella "en béret de chasseur." (b) Wiberg type III patella

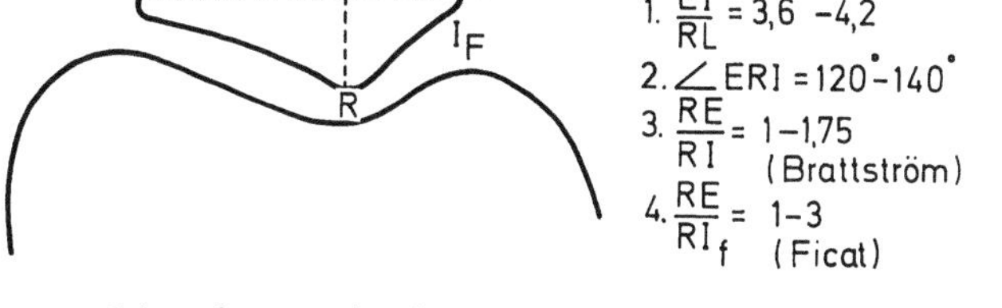

Fig. 101. Measurements according to patella type. List of normal values

Henssge (1962) found type I in 10%, type II in 65%, and type III in 25% of cases. Baumgartl (1964) found a slightly different distribution, partly because he used a different classification of patella types. He found Wiberg's type I in 11%, type II in 55%, and type III in 11% of cases, and his own type II/III in 23%. Type IV and the type *en béret de chasseur* he found to be rare. Type IV proved to be regularly associated with osteochondritis dissecans.

Many authors maintain that Wiberg's type III is an important factor in the etiology of patellar chondropathy (Gschwend, 1971; Ficat, 1970a, 1973; Fürmaier, 1953b).

Figure 101 outlines the various measurements which can be made of the patella. The patellar depth factor shows a relation between patellar width and height. Ficat (1970a) found values between 3.6 and 4.2 for this factor. He reported that angle externe-rotule-interne (ERI) averages 130° and he identifies a value of less than 110° or more than 140° with dysplasia.

The facet factor indicates the ratio between the lateral and the medial articular surface of the patella (RE:RI). Brattström (1964) regarded a value of 1–1.75 as normal. Ficat and Bizou (1967) calculated the facet factor $RE:RI_f$. This value is 1–3.

A convex shape of the medial articular surface, as in Wiberg's type III patella, is regarded by many authors as an important factor in the etiology of patellar chondropathy of the medial facet. According to Rijnks (1976), determination of angle ERI and facet factor RE:RI is sufficient, in addition to a convex medial facet, to obtain information of the structure of the patella.

Patella Partita. A patella partita is found in 0.2%–6% of all individuals (Blumensaat, 1938; Green, 1975). It is often found unilaterally (Fig. 102). In many cases a patella partita can give rise to pain, and precisely in such cases differentiation from an unhealed fracture is difficult (Smillie, 1974; Green, 1975). Ficat (1970a) and Bandi (1972) mentioned patella partita as a cause of patellar chondropathy. Rijnks (1976) maintained that a patella partita does not predispose to chondropathy.

Dysplasia of the Facies Patellaris Femoris. Dysplasia of the femoral condyles is mainly mentioned in studies of habitual luxation or subluxation of the patella (Figs. 95 and 104–107). It is almost generally accepted that underdevelopment of the lateral femoral condyle plays an important role in the etiology of patellar luxation (Brattström, 1964; Ficat, 1970a).

Brattström made very accurate measurements of the femoral condyles and maintained that the sulcus angle E′TI′ (Fig. 103)

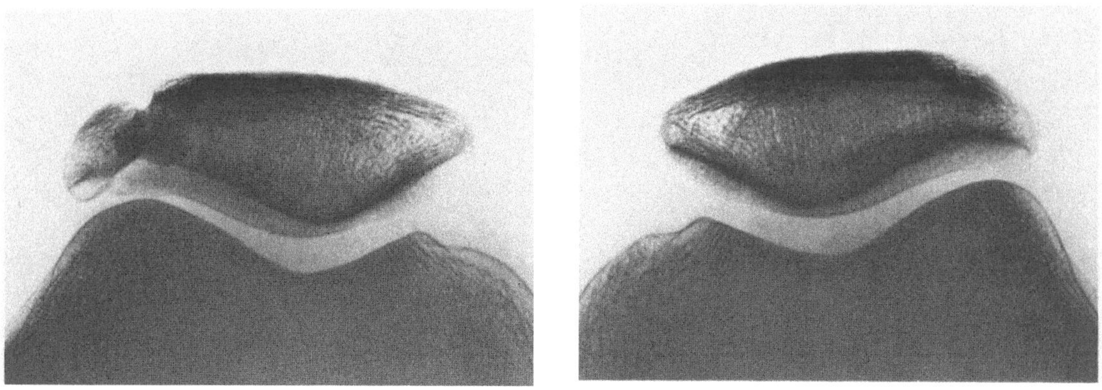

Fig. 102. Unilateral patella tripartita

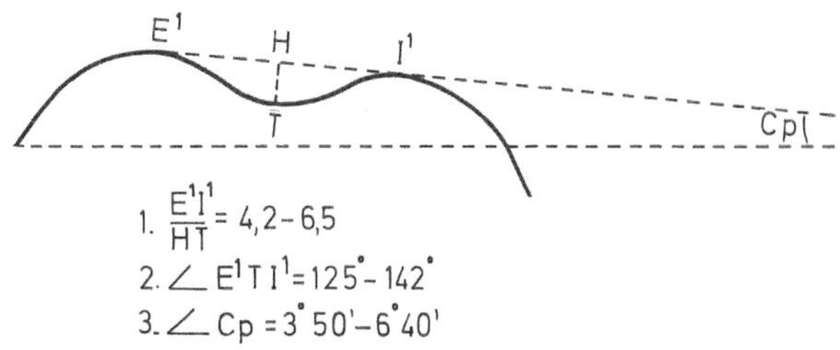

Fig. 103. Measurements of the facies patellaris femoris. Normal values

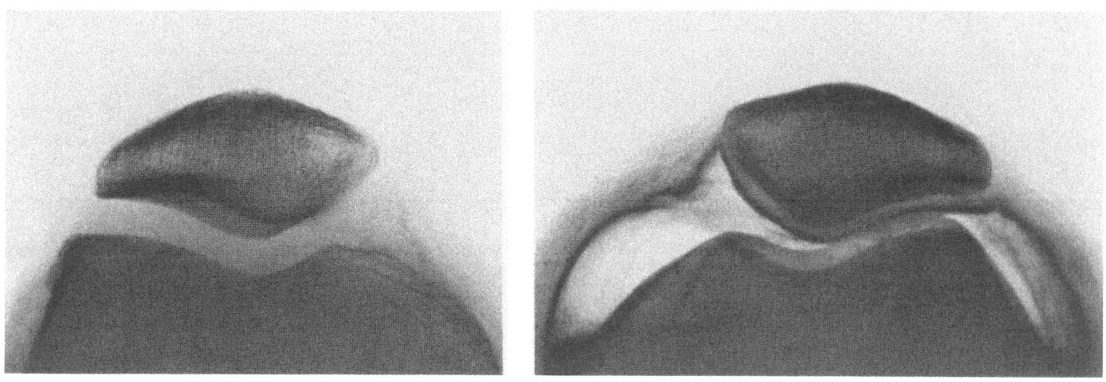

Fig. 104. Tilting of the patella and slight subluxation

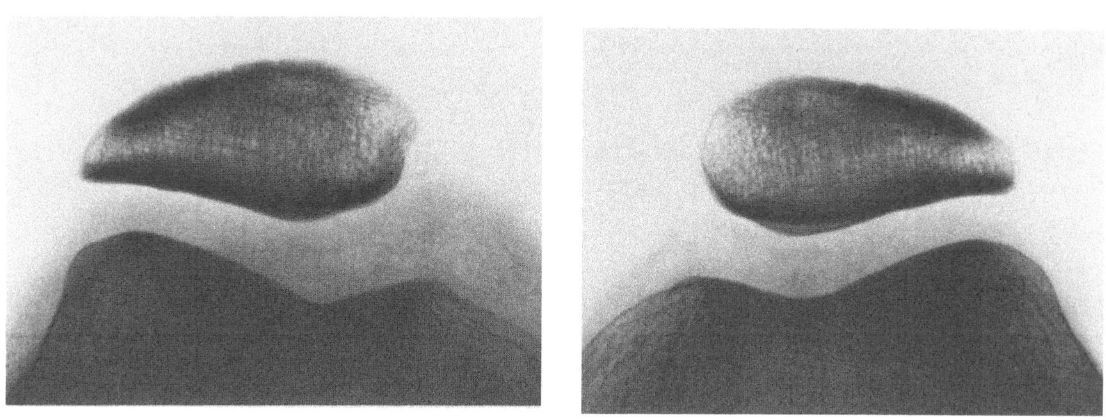

Fig. 105. Bilateral Wiberg type III patella. Left: subluxation

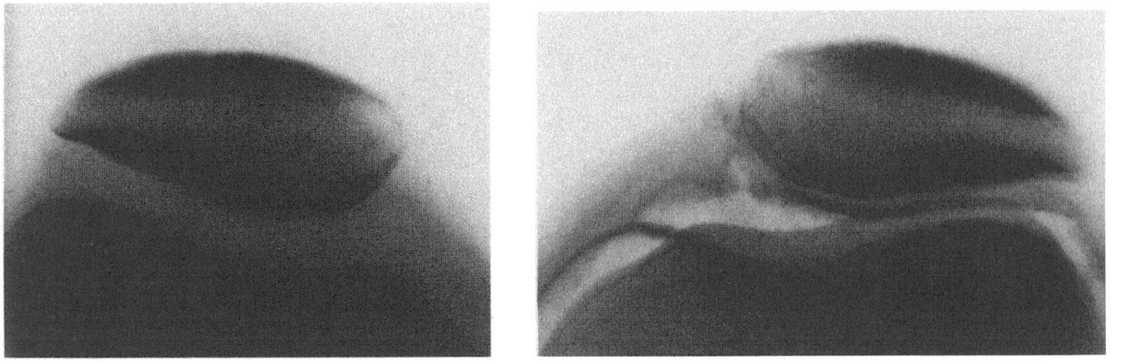

Fig. 106. Wiberg type III patella showing dysplasia and subluxation. Marked chondropathy of the patellar eminence and the medial facet

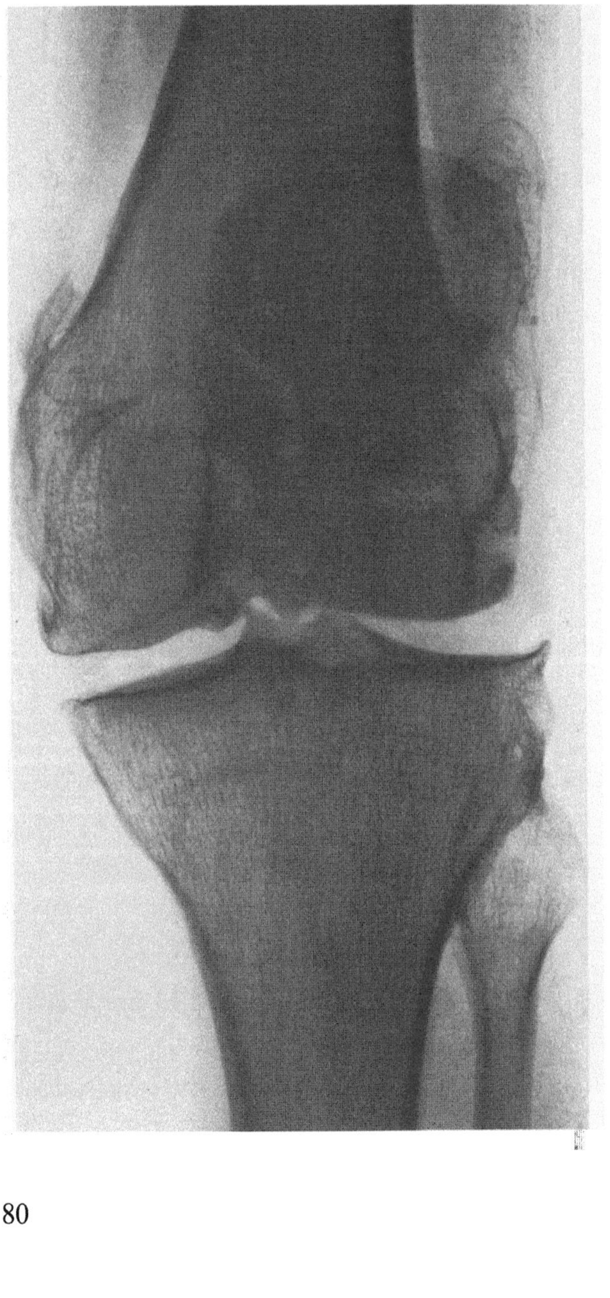

a

Fig. 107. (a–c) Luxation of the *left* patella with marked patellofemoral arthrosis and arthrotic lesions of the tibiofemoral joint. (d and e) Dysplasia of the *right* patella with lateral patellofemoral arthrosis. High patella

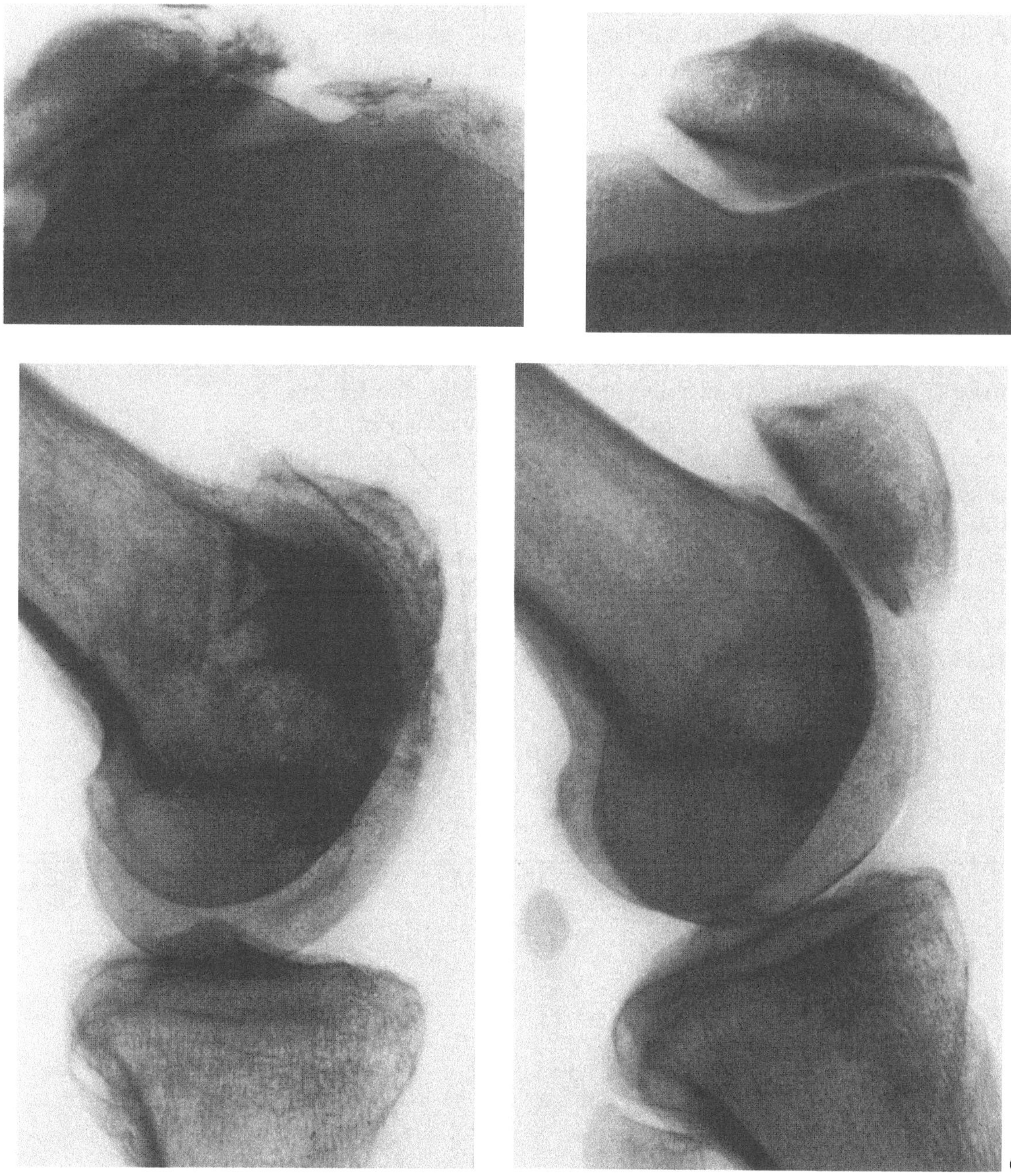

b d c e

Fig. 107. (Cont.)

gives a more precise impression of the degree of dysplasia of the femoral condyles than does the prominence of the lateral femoral condyle. This prominence is too markedly influenced by the position of the knee by tangential arthrography. Minor rotations can cause marked differences in the height of the femoral condyles, so that angle C_P (Fig. 103) can differ widely. Ficat et al. (1970b) mentioned depth factor E′I′:HT in addition to this angle. The normal ranges of variation of the various measurements are indicated in Fig. 103.

According to Rijnks (1976) there is a very close correlation between angle E′TI′ and the depth factor of the condyles. Determination of only angle E′TI′ gives insufficient information on the structure of the facies patellaris femoris.

High Patella. A high patella is a too cranially localized patella. Blumensaat (1938) measured the distance between the apex of the patella and the line through the base of the intercondylar fossa (Fig. 108) with the knee flexed 30°. Normally, the inferior pole of the patella extends as far as this line. In actual practice, accurate determination of this distance greatly depends on appropriate flexion of the knee joint. Rijnks (1976) found an average distance of 6 mm in his patients. Given highly mobile patellae and patellae with subluxation, values of 17–21 mm were found.

Insall and Salvati (1971) found that in a normal knee the length of the patellar ligament equals the length of the patella. If the length of the patellar ligament exceeds that of the patella by

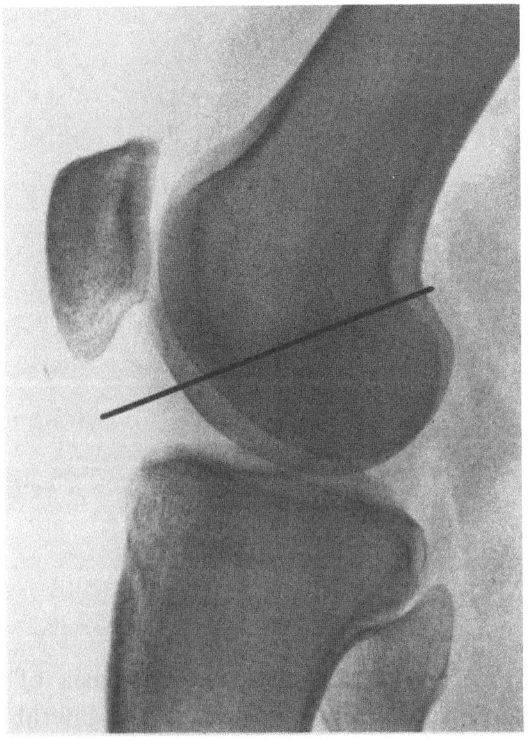

Fig. 108. Blumensaat line. The knee joint is in 30° flexion. The distance between the patellar apex and the Blumensaat line is crucial. Normal value about 6 mm. Values found in very mobile and subluxable patellae: 17–21 mm (Rijnks, 1976)

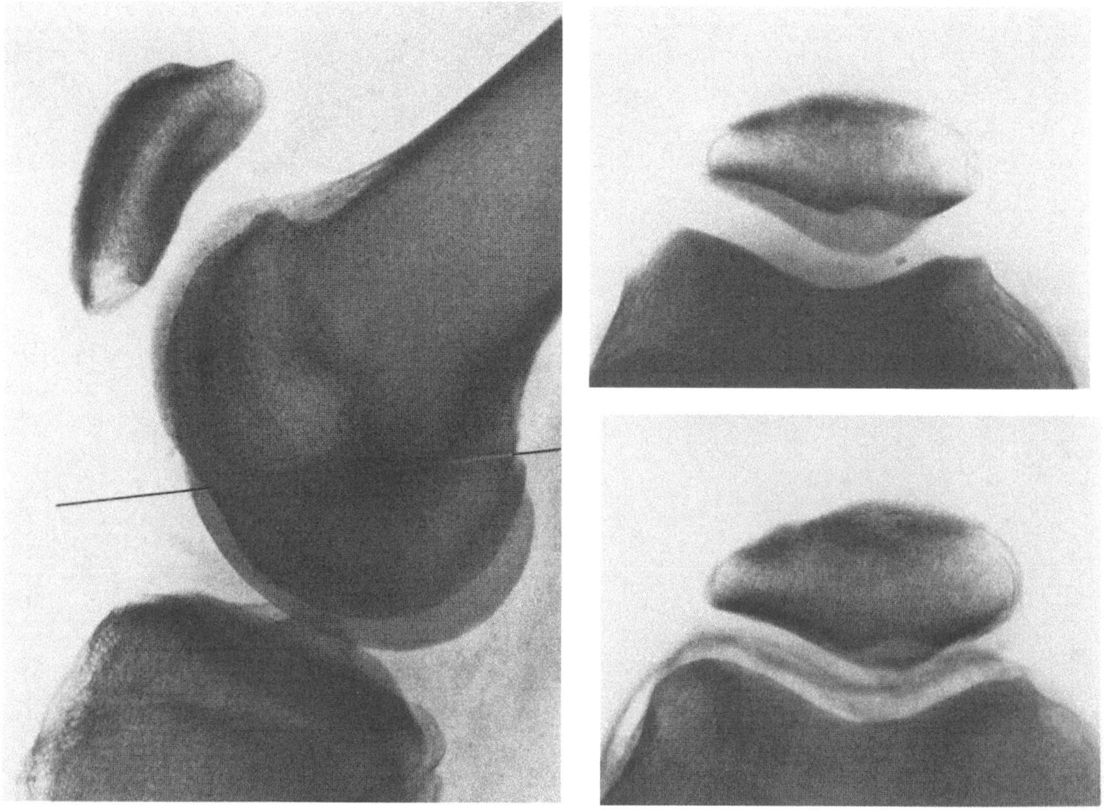

a b c

Fig. 109 a–c. Unmistakable high patella. Distance measured between patellar apex and Blumensaat line: 27 mm (a). The tangential projections clearly show structural changes, virtually conclusive of patellar chondropathy (b). Double contrast arthrography: unmistakable patellar chondropathy (c)

more than 20%, the situation is described as "high patella." The influence of a high patella on the etiology of chondropathy is explained by the incongruity of the articular surfaces in the patellofemoral joint and by marked stress within that joint. A high patella, moreover, tends to subluxate or luxate. Rijnks, too, found a positive correlation between the degree of high patella and the severity of chondropathy (Fig. 109).

Low Patella. A low patella is a too distally localized patella. It usually results from tuberosity transplantation in view of habitual patellar luxation (Fig. 110). The term low patella is used when the inferior margin of the patella is below the line through the base of the intercondylar fossa. In these cases the incongruity in the patellofemoral joint leads to patellar chondropathy.

Increased Patellar Mobility. Luxation of the patella is nearly always lateral luxation. If it is recurrent, the term habitual luxation (or subluxation) is used. Tangential projections clearly visualize the lateral dislocation of the patella in some cases. Even a 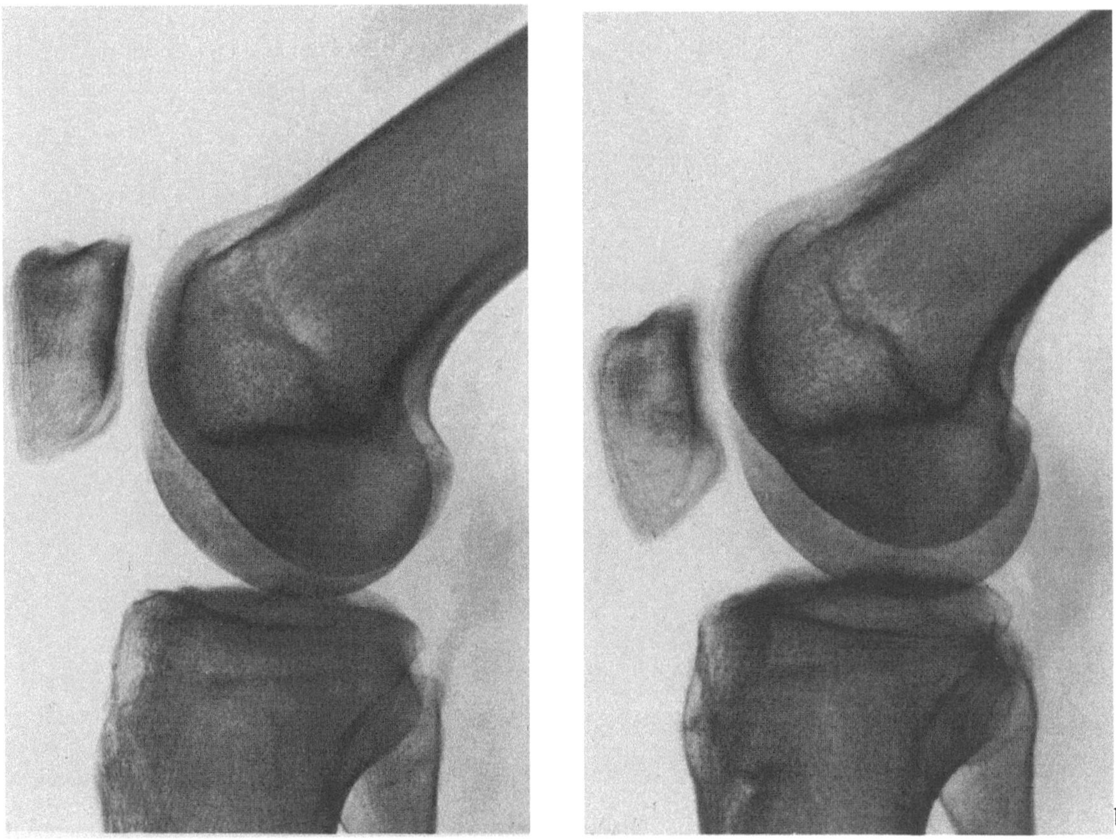 b

Fig. 110. Low patella on one side (b), due to displacement of the tibial tuberosity

slight dislocation can be observed. Ficat (1970a) diagnoses patellar subluxation if the lateral margin of the patella projects just outside the lateral femoral condyle and if the linea eminens and patellar apex also show slight lateral dislocation. Hugston (1968) distinguished a form in which the linea eminens is localized in the trochlear sulcus, but the patella is slightly tilted. This causes dilatation of the articular cavity between the medial femoral condyle and the medial articular surface of the patella. Hugston described this situation as tilting patella (Figs. 104–106). Ficat (1973) attached great importance to this tilting of the patella, maintaining that in these cases there must be increased pressure within the lateral compartment of the patellofemoral joint, which can lead to chondropathy. Subluxation or luxation of the patella involves considerable forces which can damage the cartilage. Severe patellofemoral arthrosis deformans can also be found (Fig. 107).

Patellar chondropathy and subluxation of the patella are often concomitant. In many cases, patellar chondropathy is even believed to be a result of habitual subluxation of the patella, as Rijnks (1976) observed in all cases of luxation or subluxation. The causes of (sub)luxation of the patella may lie in a lateral traction resultant of the quadriceps femoris muscle which is not in line with the patellar ligament. This produces a lateral force which has a luxating effect on the patella. Other possible causes of (sub)luxation are a flaccid joint capsule or shrinking of the lateral part of the joint capsule. In addition, high patella or patellar dysplasia can be etiologic factors.

Increased Pressure in the Patellofemoral Joint. The force which presses the patella against the femur is greatly increased by flexion of the knee joint. The stress involved in walking stairs can amount to 2–3 times the body weight. Maximum values of 8–13 times the body weight can be found during squatting on one leg. In a normal knee joint, the increase in compressive force is not always present; an increase occurs only at flexion. A permanent increase in compressive force leads to a continuously increased pressure between patella and femoral condyles. This can give rise to arthrosis. An indication of this increased pressure can be found in osteosclerosis at the site of the increased pressure. Maquet (1976) clearly demonstrated the course of thc lines of force in synthetic models. The syndrome that involves increased pressure especially in the lateral part of the patellofemoral joint was described by Ficat (1970) as *le syndrome d'hyperpression externe de la rotule*. The cause of this increased pressure is lateral tilting of the patella. Such a syndrome can readily develop in the case of subluxation (Figs. 104 and 105). Radiographs can show a tilting patella as well as calcification in the lateral retinaculum. In addition, there is increased density of the subchondral bone of the lateral patellar facet and narrowing of the lateral patellofemoral articular cavity.

4.3.3 Non-Mechanical Lesions of the Patellar Cartilage

Systemic diseases which can lead to non-mechanical lesions of the patellar cartilage include rheumatoid arthritis and hemophilia. These conditions can lead to total destruction of the knee joint (Fig. 111). It seems likely that changes which occur after a knee injury, arthrotomy or immobilization in a plaster cast, exert an influence on the development of a chondropathy. Disorders of cartilage nutrition as a result of the absent pump mechanism may also play a role. A lesion or decreased resistance of the cartilage can result. In this context hydrops, post-traumatic dystrophy, and hemarthros also seem to be important (Fig. 112).

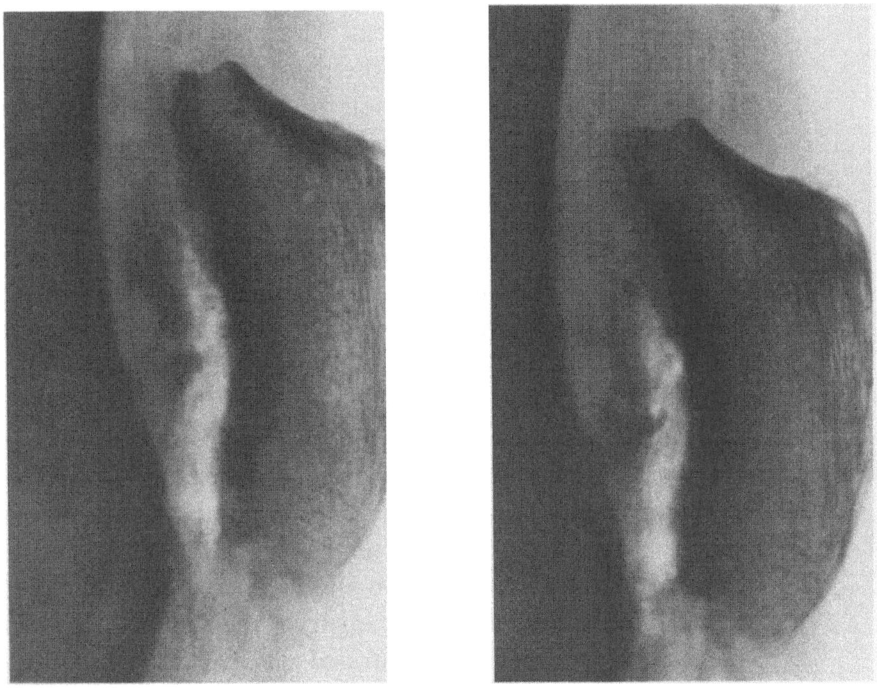

Fig. 111. Rheumatoid arthritis. Marked destruction of the retropatellar cartilage. Severe synovitis

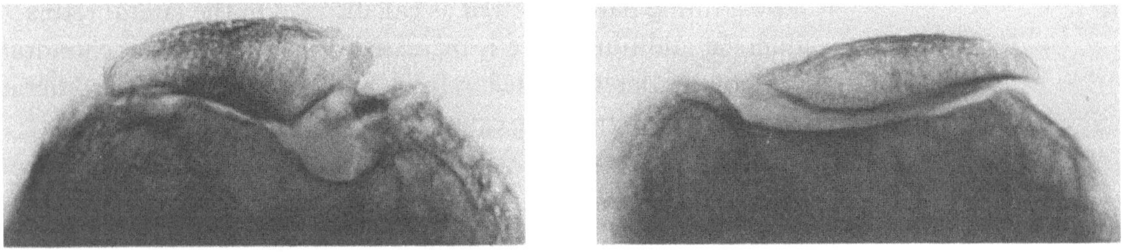

Fig. 112. Hemophilia. Marked deformation of the patellofemoral joint in both knees

4.4. Radiologic Diagnosis of Patellar Chondropathy

The preceding sections of this chapter have already discussed the factors in the etiology of patellar chondropathy. The changes found in patellar chondropathy will be based on radiographs taken without injection of contrast medium and on double contrast arthrograms.

4.4.1 Radiologic Examination Without Contrast Medium

Particularly in early stages of chondropathy, skeletal changes need not be present. Sclerosis of the lateral patellar facet and a narrowed articular cavity indicate increased pressure between the lateral patellar facet and the lateral femoral condyle (Figs. 104 and 105). Chondropathy is frequently present in such cases. In many cases of chondropathy the posterior aspect of the patella shows slight subchondral decalcification, which in some cases can lead to an irregular defect in the posterior osseous boundary of the patella, particularly on the linea eminens (Figs. 109 and 113). Small exostoses are often visible on the posterior margins of the patella (Fig. 114). These are usually visible in lateral as well as in tangential projections and can be indicative of patellar chondropathy.

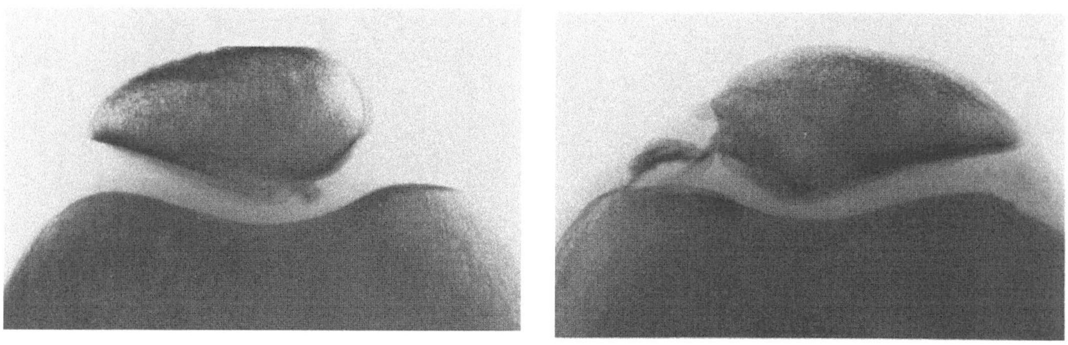

Fig. 113. Marfan's disease: bilateral habitual patellar luxation. Marked structural changes in both patellae. Right knee: calcifications in the patellar retinaculum. Bilateral patellar dysplasia (Wiberg type III)

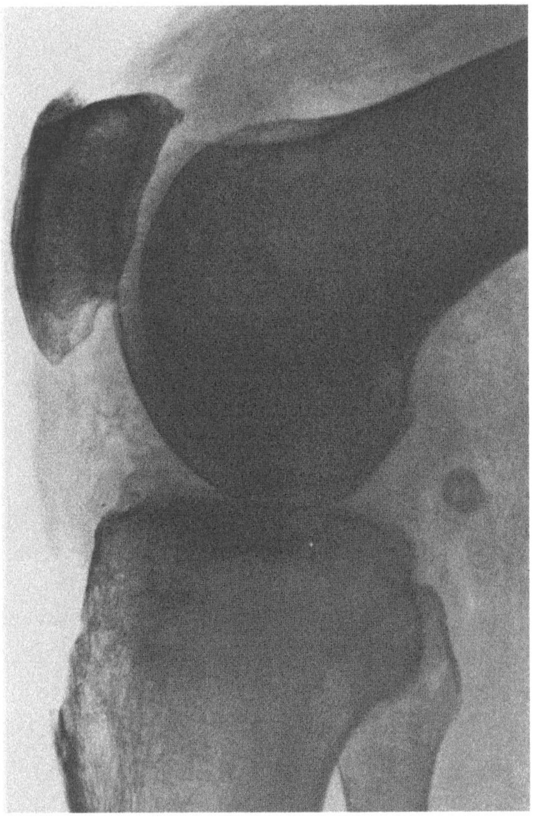

Fig. 114. Skeletal lesions in patellar chondropathy. Slight structural changes in the patella and incipient hook formation

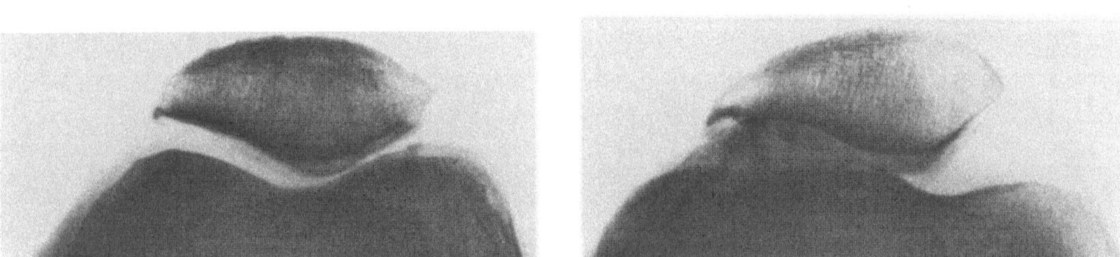

Fig. 115. Bilateral patellofemoral arthrosis. Right radiograph: subluxation

Marked narrowing of the patellofemoral articular cavity, structural changes, and hook formation are features of arthrosis deformans. It should be remembered that patellar chondropathy is merely a preliminary stage of arthrosis, not a separate entity. As already described, there is an increased risk of patellar chondropathy in the case of tilting, (sub)luxation, or dysplasia of the patella (Figs. 104–107 and 115).

4.4.2 Double Contrast Arthrography

In the lateral projection the thickness of the retropatellar cartilage is normally 4–5 mm at the maximum. Although incipient chondropathy can initially cause swelling of the cartilage, most cases show a reduced thickness of retropatellar cartilage. This need not involve the entire cartilage surface but can be very circumscribed. Lateral as well as tangential projections of the patella often clearly demonstrate the reduced thickness of the cartilage (Figs. 116, 117, and 120). Maldague and Malghem (1976) photographed separately the medial and the lateral facet of the patella in lateral projection. We have also used this method. Superposi-

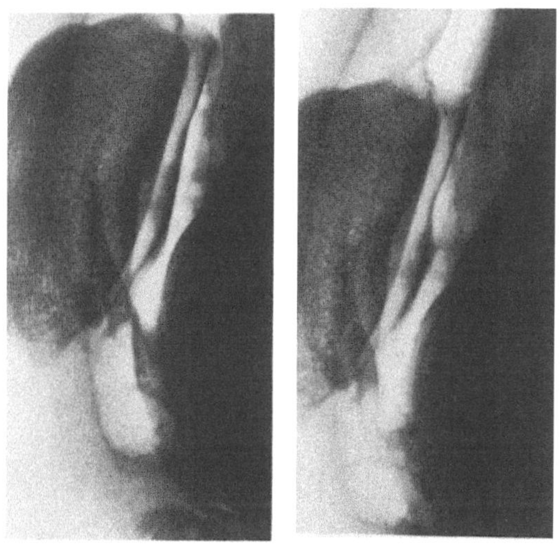

Fig. 116. Situation after lateral meniscectomy. Double contrast arthrography: narrowing of the retropatellar cartilage due to patellar chondropathy

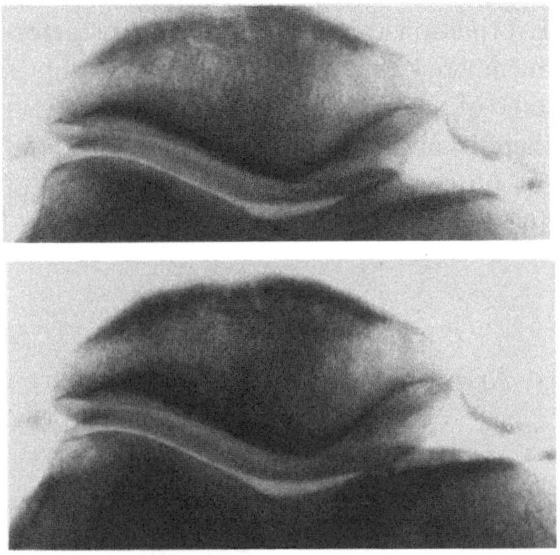

Fig. 117. Patellar chondropathy at the linea eminens, characterized by narrowing of the layer of cartilage

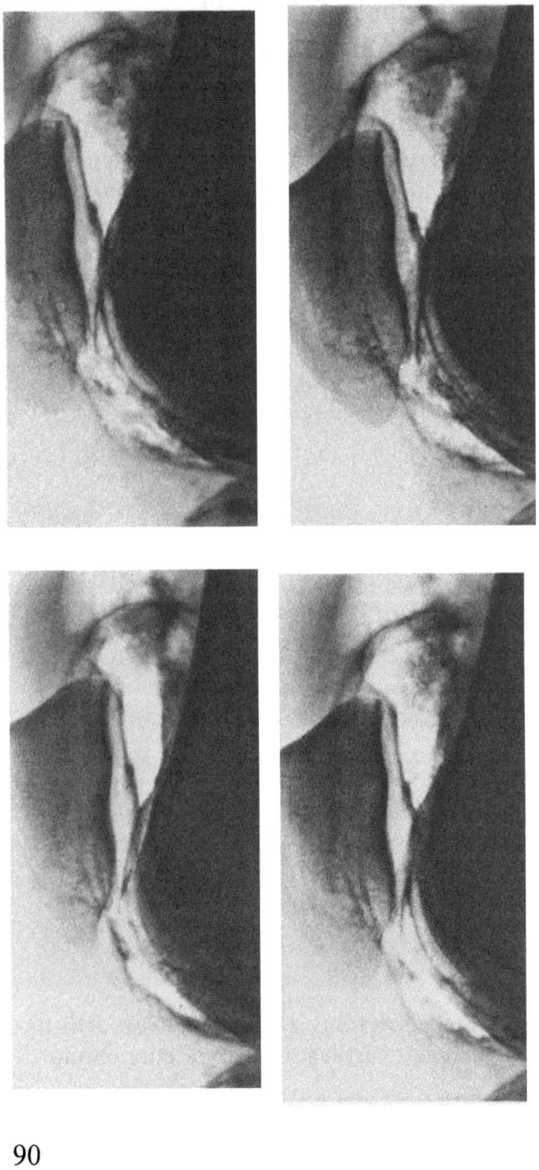

Fig. 118. Arthrography in lateral direction. Irregular posterior delimitation of the patella due to patellar chondropathy

Fig. 119. Patellar dysplasia. Large, flat patella; large angle ERI. Arthrography: distinctly small and irregularly defined retropatellar cartilage. Patellar chondropathy

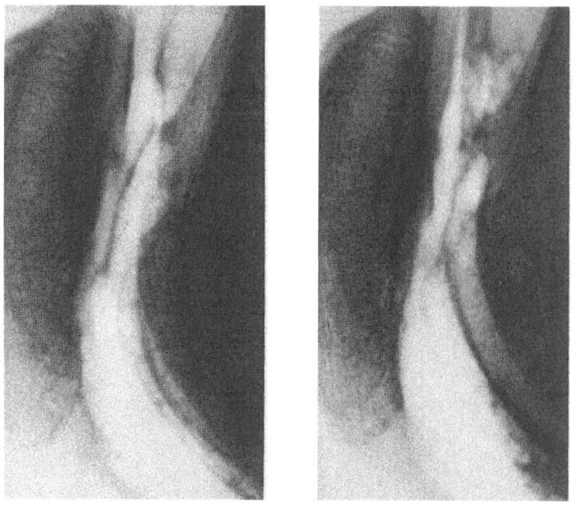

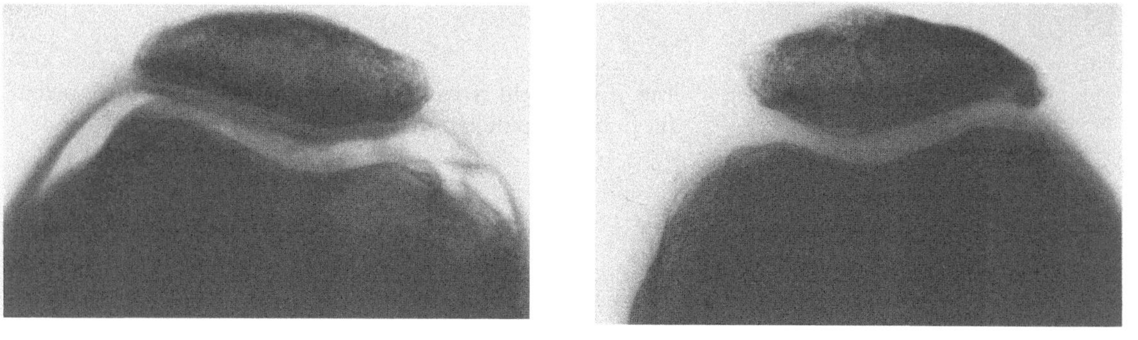

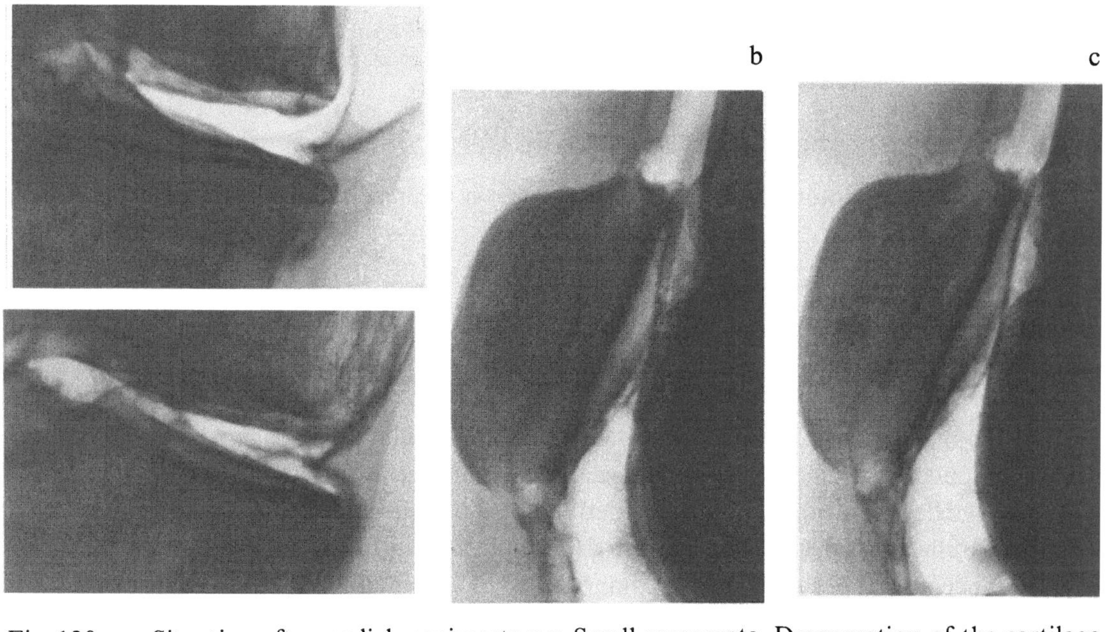

a

b

c

Fig. 120a–c. Situation after medial meniscectomy. Small regenerate. Degeneration of the cartilage of femur and tibial plateau (a). Narrowing and irregular inferior delimitation of the retropatellar cartilage. Patellar chondropathy (b and c)

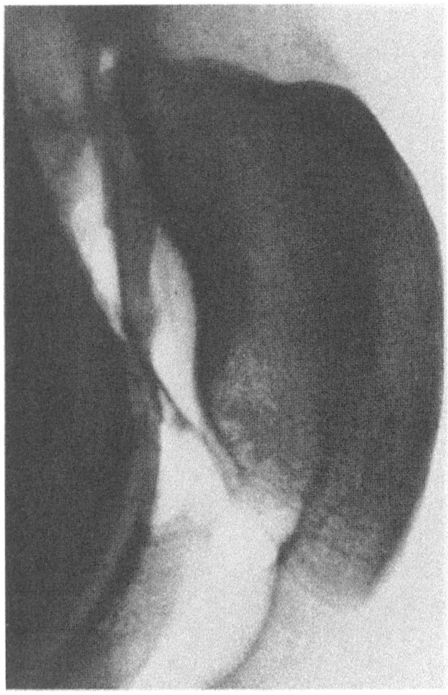

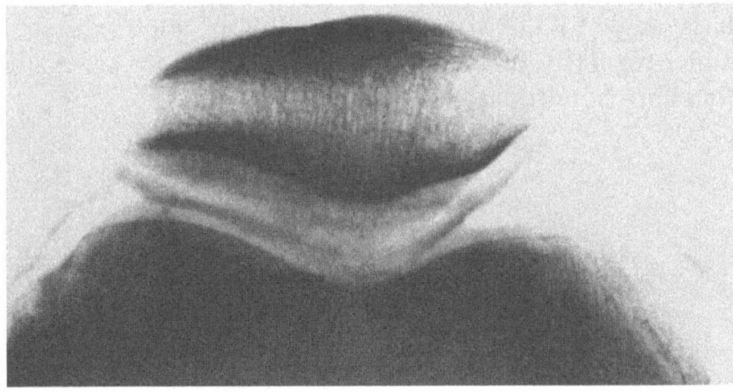

Fig. 121. Slight irregularity of the cartilage on the medial facet. Slight patellar chondropathy

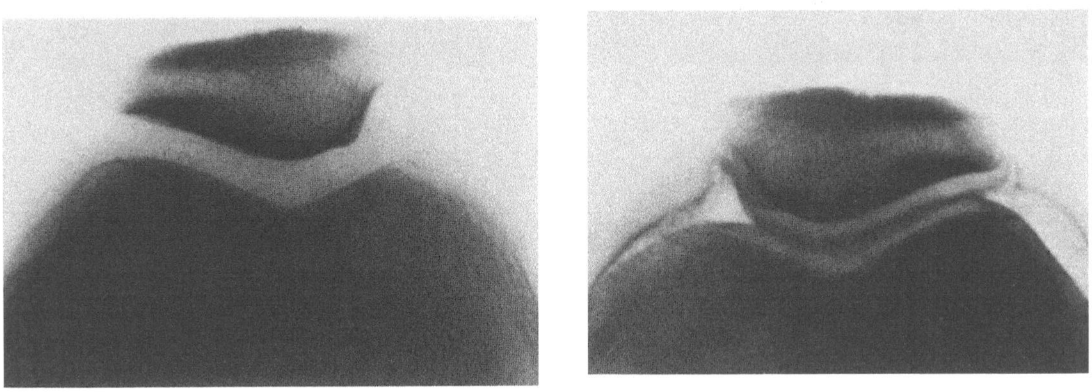

Fig. 122. Irregular contour of the patellar cartilage on the medial facet. Patellar chondropathy

tion of the femoral condyles impedes evaluation of these radiographs, and the results are therefore less reliable, in our opinion.

Apart from reduction of the thickness of the retropatellar cartilage, irregular cartilage contours are demonstrable as a result of cartilage degeneration. The sharply defined posterior boundary of the patella disappears. The posterior delimitation is blurred instead because the superficial cartilage layer is imbibed with contrast medium (Figs. 118 and 119). In some cases the changes are still very slight: only some irregularity of the retropatellar cartilage, still without marked reduction of its thickness

(Figs. 121 and 122). Not always do lateral and tangential projections reveal the changes, in some cases it is the lateral, in other cases the tangential projections that reveal most changes. This applies in particular to the milder forms of patellar chondropathy.

4.5 Correlation Between Double Contrast Arthrography and Arthroscopy

The reliability of arthrographic diagnosis was studied in a group of 216 patients examined first by arthrography and then by arthroscopy. Of the 135 patients in whom arthrography revealed no lesion of the retropatellar cartilage, 96 (71%) showed a positive correlation with the arthroscopic findings (Table 5); in the remaining 39 patients, arthrography proved to be false negative (29%).

The arthrographic diagnosis of patellar chondropathy proved to be correct in 67 of the 81 patients (83%). A false positive result was obtained in 14 patients (17%) (Table 5).

Of the false negative results obtained in 39 patients with patellar chondropathy, 29 were based on slight degenerative changes (grades I and I/II). Grade II proved to exist in 8 patients, and grade II/III in 2. The severe grade III and IV were always correctly diagnosed (Table 6).

Table 5. Correlation between double contrast arthrography and arthroscopy in patellar chondropathy

Arthrography	Pos. correlation arthrography–arthroscopy	False neg. arthrogram	False pos. arthrogram	Number of patients
No abnormalities	96 (71%)	39 (29%)	–	135
Patellar chondropathy	67 (83%)	–	14 (17%)	81
				216

Table 6. False negative arthrographic diagnosis in 39 patients with patellar chondropathy; this false negative diagnosis was made chiefly in grades I and I/II

Arthroscopy	
Grade I	17
Grade I–II	12
Grade II	8
Grade II–III	2
Grade III	–
Grade III–IV	–
Grade IV	–
Number of patients	39

If we eliminate the arthrographic diagnosis "no lesions" in the tables and base ourselves on the arthroscopic diagnosis "patellar chondropathy," the accuracy of arthrography proves to be much lower (Table 7).

Butt (1969) found an accuracy of double contrast arthrography of only about 50% in patellar chondropathy, and his false negative results likewise concerned the still mild forms of chondropathy.

In the tables it is presumed that the arthroscopist diagnosed patellar chondropathy with 100% accuracy. The grade of chondropathy found by the arthroscopist varied widely. Table 8 indicates the grade of cartilage degeneration (cf. Sect. 4.2.4) in the 106 patients of Table 5 in whom the arthroscopist diagnosed patellar chondropathy.

Although double contrast arthrography is not optimally accurate in the diagnosis of patellar chondropathy, the severe grades of

Table 7. Correlation between double contrast arthrography and arthroscopy in 120 patients in whom patellar chondropathy had been arthroscopically diagnosed with certainty

	Arthrography		Arthroscopy	
Correct +	67	56%	120	100% (?)
Dubious	–	–	–	–
False +	14	12%	–	–
False –	39	32%	–	–
Total	120		120	

Table 8. Severity of patellar chondropathy as established at arthroscopy. Comparison with Table 6 leads to the conclusion that the severe grades of patellar chondropathy can be readily diagnosed arthrographically

Arthroscopy	
Grade I	37
Grade I–II	23
Grade II	19
Grade II–III	9
Grade III	7
Grade III–IV	7
Grade IV	4
Number of patients	106

chondropathy were all correctly diagnosed. The minor changes in the initial stage of the degeneration, characterized by only some maceration of patellar cartilage while the contours are not yet very irregular, are of course not demonstrable with certainty.

5 Cruciate Ligaments

5.1 Anatomy of the Cruciate Ligaments

The anterior cruciate ligament is proximally connected to the inside of the lateral femoral condyle in the intercondylar fossa. In its more distal course the cruciate ligament is slightly narrower, and attached to the tibial plateau in an area medio-anterior to the intercondylar eminence, between the sites of insertion of the two menisci (Fig. 9). A number of fibers of the anterior cruciate ligament often connect to the anterior horn of the medial meniscus. As a result, rupture of the anterior cruciate ligament is regularly associated with a lesion of the medial meniscus. The anterior cruciate ligament is completely taut at maximum extension and maximally relaxed at 20° flexion of the knee joint. When flexion is continued, the cruciate ligament is gradually tautened until the knee joint attains 120° flexion. The posterior cruciate ligament lies behind the anterior cruciate ligament, decussates with it and is slightly stronger. This cruciate ligament fans out proximally to connect to the medial inside of the intercondylar fossa and then narrows down to extend obliquely in a direction distal to the fibula. It inserts in the posterior tibial intercondylar fossa and on the posterior aspect of the tibia, dorsal to the sites of insertion of the two posterior meniscal horns. The meniscifibular ligament consists of a narrow bundle of fibers connecting the posterior horn of the lateral meniscus to the posterior cruciate ligament. This ligament takes its course dorsal to the posterior cruciate ligament (Fig. 123).

As a result of their anatomic structure and fixation, the two cruciate ligaments decussate. The decussation is such that the cruciate ligaments move slightly apart at exorotation and then relax. Endorotation is inhibited because the cruciate ligaments are slightly twisted together. Both ligaments are connected to each other and to the posterior joint capsule by low-density connective tissue, adipose tissue, and vessels.

Motion studies have demonstrated that the cruciate ligaments permanently control the flexion-and-extension movements in the

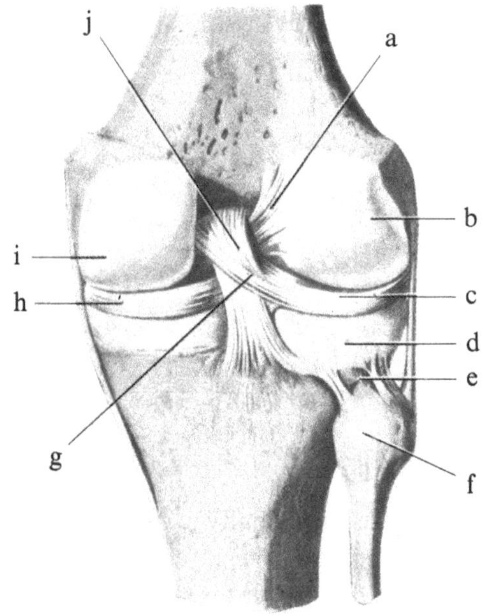

Fig. 123. Posterior view of the right knee joint (after W. Spalteholz, 1954) *a*. Ligamentum cruciatum anterius; *b*. Condylus lateralis femoris; *c*. Meniscus lateralis; *d*. Facies poplitea tibiae; *e*. Articulatio tibiofibularis; *f*. Capitulum fibulae; *g*. Ligamentum meniscifibularis; *h*. Meniscus medialis; *i*. Condylus medialis femoris; *j*. Ligamentum cruciatum posterius

knee joint, because these movements always tauten part of the anterior as well as part of the posterior cruciate ligaments. In flexion of the knee, the two opposite parts of the cruciate ligaments prove to tauten, while in extension it is precisely the parts of the ligaments not in contact with each other that are tautened. This means that with the knee extended, the anterior half of the anterior cruciate ligament and the posterior half of the posterior cruciate ligament are tautened (Spalteholz, 1954). The tautness of the anterior cruciate ligament increases as flexion of the knee joint increases. The ligament is maximally tautened in extension and at 120° flexion.

Fibers of the posterior cruciate ligament are tautened throughout the arc of flexion. With increasing extension, the function of the posterior cruciate ligament increases (Fischer et al., 1978).

Owing to their particular course, the cruciate ligaments are of great importance to the stability of the knee joint (not only for anteroposterior but also for lateral stability). Rupture of the anterior cruciate ligament leads to excessive anterior mobility of the tibia. With simultaneous lesion of the medial collateral ligament, moreover, anteromedial mobility in the joint can also increase. In such cases it is easy to dilate the medial articular

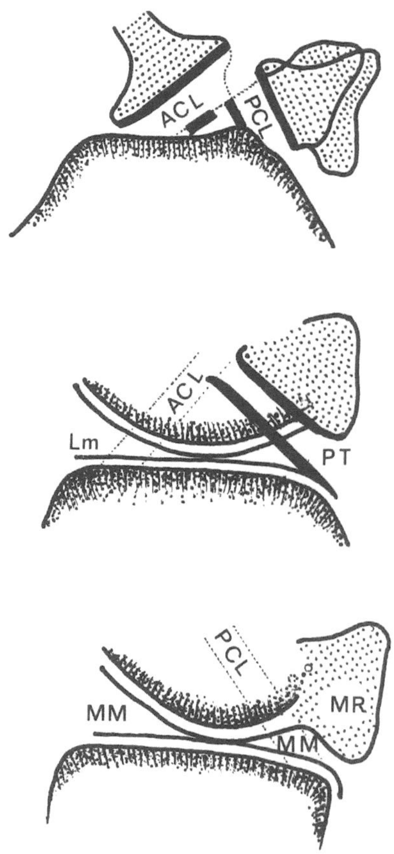

Fig. 125. Diagrams of arthrographically visible parts of both cruciate ligaments (after Lindblom, 1938). ACL anterior cruciate ligament; PCL posterior cruciate ligament; PT Popliteal tendon; LM Lateral meniscus; MM Medial meniscus; MR Medial recess of the articular cavity behind the medial condyle

cavity by exerting mediolateral pressure on the tibia. Rupture of the posterior cruciate ligament leads to excessive posterior mobility of the tibia. The anterior cruciate ligament is clearly visible by arthroscopy (Fig. 124 see page 143).

On the anterior side, the synovial membrane continues onto the anterior cruciate ligament, and covers its lateral and anterior aspects over virtually the entire length. The synovial membrane is generally absent on the medial side at the level of decussation with the posterior cruciate ligament, unless the synovial membrane protrudes between the two cruciate ligaments.

The synovial membrane as a rule covers only a small part of the posterior aspect of the anterior cruciate ligament, but in some cases a larger part may be lined. Arthrography can depict only those parts of the cruciate ligaments that are covered by the synovial membrane (Fig. 125) (Lindblom, 1938; Liljedahl et al., 1966).

At its insertion on the femoral condyle, the posterior cruciate ligament is in virtually circular contact with the articular cavity. On the posterior side of the joint, the synovial membrane forms a large recess around both femoral condyles. On the posterior side of the cruciate ligament the medial recess extends distally as far as the superior surface of the medial meniscus. This is why most of the length of the posterior contour of the posterior cruciate ligament can be depicted. A small part of the anterior contour of the cruciate ligament usually is also visible. In some patients, both the posterior contour of the anterior cruciate ligament and the anterior contour of the posterior cruciate ligament can be visible over virtually their entire length, if a marked protrusion of the synovial membrane between the cruciate ligaments is present.

The above clearly shows that both cruciate ligaments are localized outside the synovial membrane and therefore outside the capsule. Together with the infrapatellar synovial fold, the cruciate ligaments are regarded as remnants of a fetal vertical and sagittal division of the knee joint.

5.2 Radiologic Technique

As in the diagnosis of meniscal lesions, both single contrast arthrography with a positive contrast medium and double contrast arthrography are in use in the diagnosis of cruciate ligament lesions. According to Liljedahl (1966) and Fagerberg (1956), single contrast arthrography should be most accurate. However, we have not used this technique because we believe that evaluation of the menisci and the retropatellar cartilage is more difficult this way.

As part of normal double contrast arthrography, a good impression of the cruciate ligaments can be had in lateral projection with the knee joint flexed. Most authors flex the knee joint 60°–90° (Liljedahl et al., 1966; Staple, 1972; Fischedick, 1971).

Since the various parts of the anterior cruciate ligament are taut during extension and 120° flexion, lateral projection of the anterior cruciate ligament in these positions ought to be preferred. Parts of the posterior cruciate ligament are taut throughout the arc of flexion. The tautness of the posterior cruciate ligament increases with increasing extension of the knee joint (Fischer et al., 1978).

At 90° flexion, therefore, both the anterior and the posterior cruciate ligament show some degree of tautness. This is why we examine the patient with the knee flexed 90°. The anterior and the posterior cruciate ligaments are tautened by traction and pressure on the lower leg, respectively (cf. Sect. 2.3).

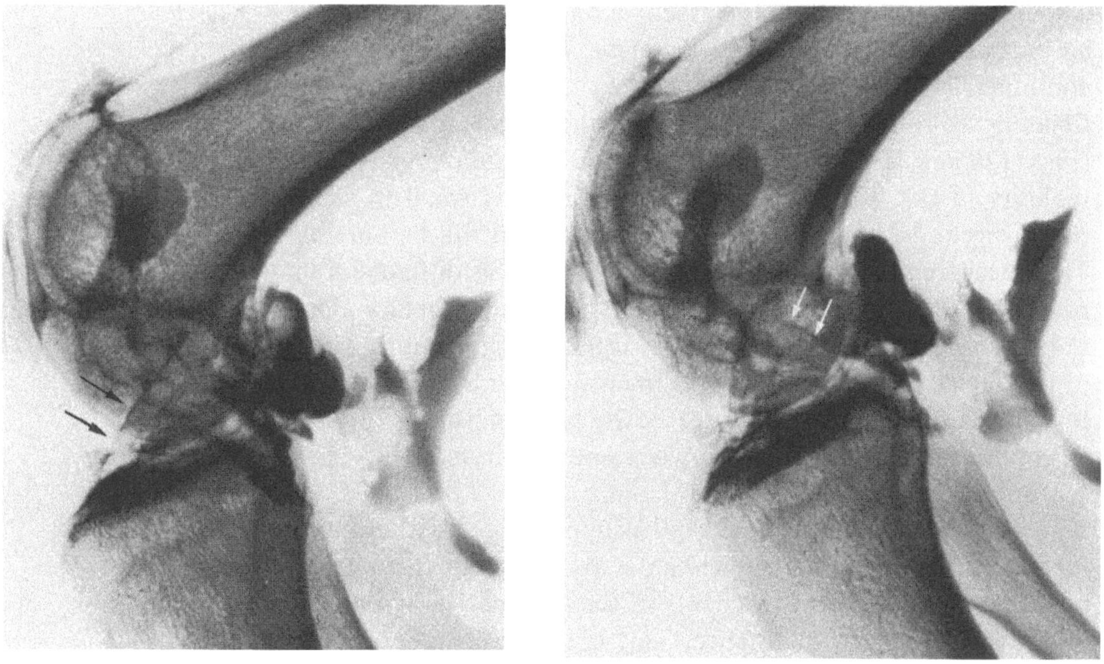

Fig. 126. Normal depiction of both cruciate ligaments (*arrows*). Large semimembranosogastrocnemial bursa

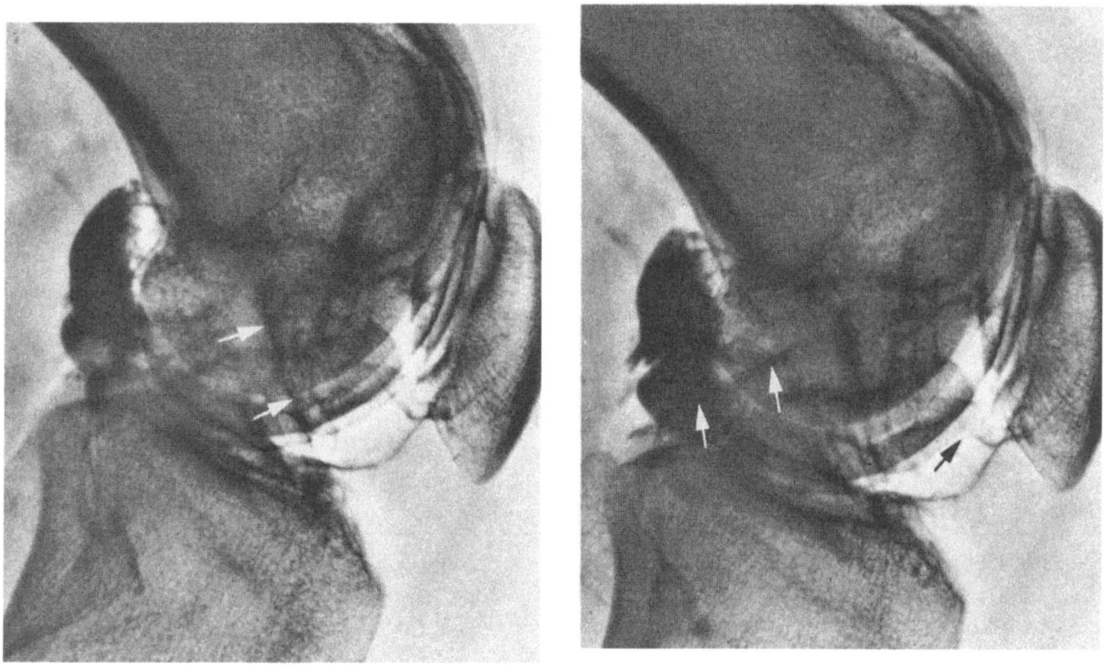

Fig. 127. Normal depiction of both cruciate ligaments (*white arrows*). Clearly visible infrapatellar synovial fold (*black arrow*)

The projection during ventral traction on the lower leg reveals an extended anterior cruciate ligament with a sharp anterior contour. The second projection, during dorsal pressure on the tibia, reveals the posterior cruciate ligament compartment (Figs. 126 and 127). With the knee joint adequately relaxed, the mobility of the tibia in relation to the femur is small in these two projections. A displacement of 5–10 mm can still be normal. This measurement, however, can be impeded by differences in rotation of the lower leg. Moreover, increased mobility does not always mean the presence of a cruciate ligament rupture; in protracted hydrops, too, the ligaments can be hyperextended. In clinical examination, therefore, the drawer sign (*vordere Schublade*) of both knees is compared when anterior cruciate ligament rupture is suspected.
If necessary, lateral projections can be supplemented with tomography (Mittler et al., 1972; Dalinka et al., 1976). In the anteroposterior projections the ligaments of the knee can be visualized only over a very short distance. This is why we make no use of these projections.
Double contrast arthrography combined with xerography might further improve diagnosis by contrast enhancement on the surfaces of the cruciate ligaments (Griffiths et al., 1974). The cruciate ligaments have recently been examined by computerized axial tomography (Pavlov et al., 1977; Archer et al., 1978), but this method seems too expensive for routine use.

5.3 Radiologic Anatomy of the Cruciate Ligaments

5.3.1 Anterior Cruciate Ligament

The anterior contour of the anterior cruciate ligament extends to about 1 cm behind the anterior margin of the tibial plateau. The ligament is extended when ventral traction is applied to the tibia. The anterior contour of the ligament is depicted as

▷

Fig. 130. Depiction of the anterior cruciate ligament. The posterior aspect of the anterior cruciate ligament is evidently formed by the recess behind the lateral femoral condyle (*arrows*)

Fig. 131. Depiction of the anterior cruciate ligament. Fluid level ventral to the ligament

Fig. 128 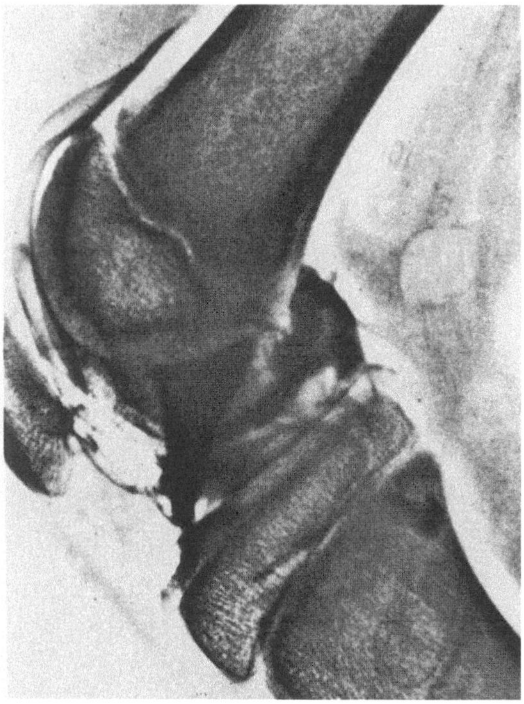 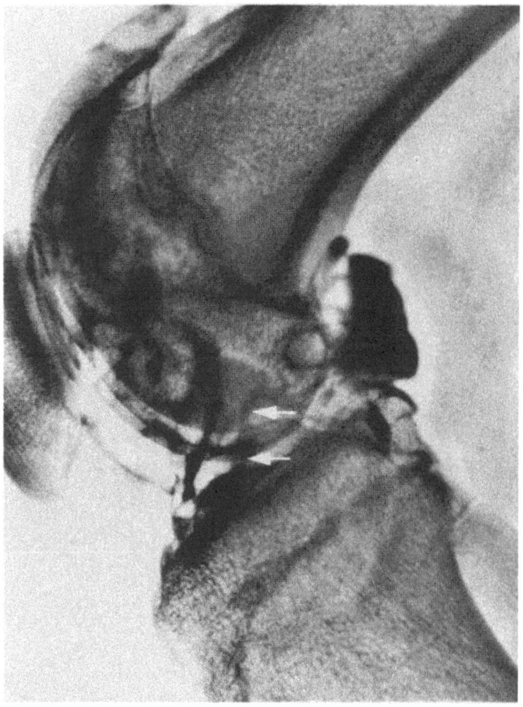 Fig. 129

Fig. 128. Course of anterior cruciate ligament. Transition from ligament to intercondylar fossa relatively far dorsally. Fluid level ventral to the cruciate ligament

Fig. 129. Posterior delimitation of the anterior cruciate ligament near the tibial plateau (*arrows*)

Fig. 130 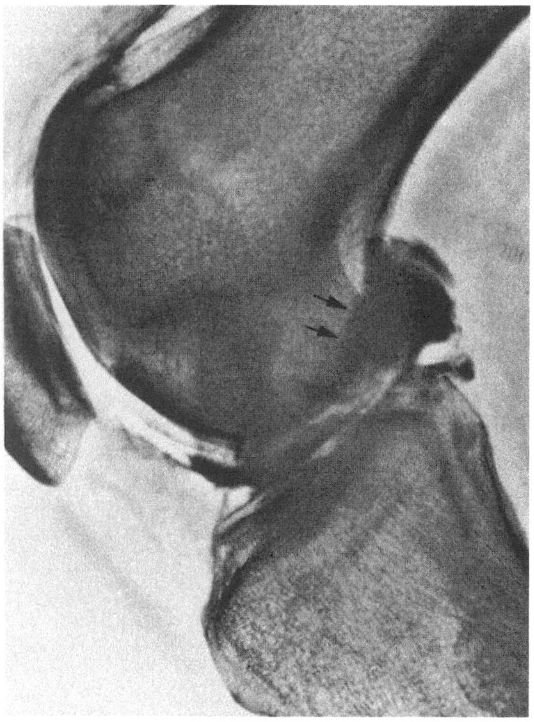 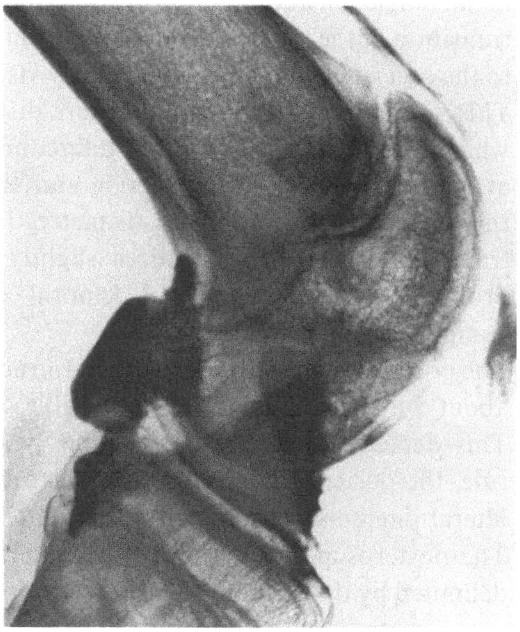 Fig. 131

Fig. 132 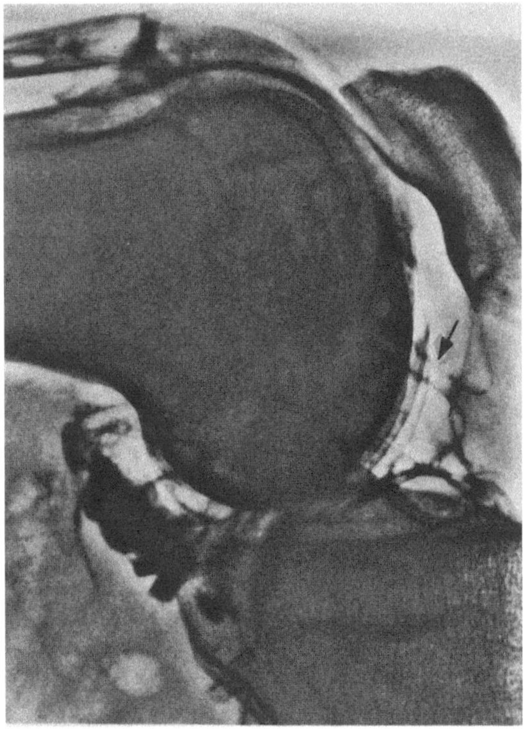 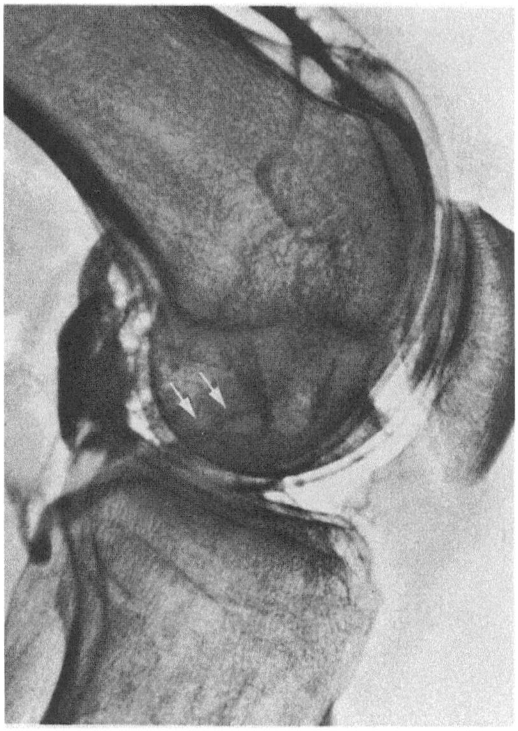 Fig. 13:

Fig. 132. Depiction of the infrapatellar synovial fold (*arrow*)

Fig. 133. Anterior delimitation of the posterior cruciate ligament (*arrows*) more clearly visible than the posterior delimitation

a straight line, projected obliquely over the femoral condyles at an angle of about 45° with the tibial plateau. The site of transition of the synovial membrane from the intercondylar fossa to the cruciate ligament is often clearly visible (Figs. 126 and 127). This site is usually a few millimeters distal to the sclerotic line which indicates the floor of the intercondylar fossa and roughly at a point between the posterior and the middle one-third of the anteroposterior condylar diameter. In juvenile subjects this transition seems to be localized slightly more dorsally; this is probably because the distal femoral epiphysis has not yet completed its growth (Fig. 128).

The posterior contour of the anterior cruciate ligament, normally about 5 mm thick, is not always visible, as already pointed out. This depends on the course of the synovial membrane. As a rule, the posterior contour is demonstrable at the base near the lateral intercondylar eminence (Figs. 127 and 129).

The posterosuperior aspect of the anterior cruciate ligament is delimited by the roof of the large recess localized on the posterior side of the lateral femoral condyle (Figs. 127 and 130). The midportion of the posterior contour of the anterior cruciate ligament (where it decussates with the posterior cruciate ligament) is not visualized.

A seemingly sharp delimitation of the anterior cruciate ligament can be caused by a fluid level in the anterior compartment of the joint. This fluid level is the interface between the contrast medium injected (sometimes mixed with synovial fluid which has remained behind) and air. With the patient in a sitting position this fluid level, like the cruciate ligament, can form an angle with the tibial plateau and thus be mistaken for a contour of the anterior cruciate ligament (Figs. 128, 130, 131, and 139). It should be remembered, however, that the anterior cruciate ligament should be depicted as a filling defect in the contrast medium behind the sharp anterior delimitation. This is why differentiation from such a fluid level offers little difficulty in most cases. Moreover, the anterior delimitation of the anterior cruciate ligament is often visible despite the spurious image.

Another configuration in the anterior compartment of the joint that can imitate an anterior cruciate ligament contour is the image of the infrapatellar synovial fold (Dalinka et al., 1976), which connects the Hoffa body to the intercondylar fossa. This ligament largely consists of a synovial fold which contains adipose tissue. Differentiation from the anterior cruciate ligament is not difficult, however, because the synovial fold takes a much more ventral course, while the anterior cruciate ligament can usually be clearly followed as far as the tibial plateau (Figs. 12, 132, and 133).

5.3.2 Posterior Cruciate Ligament

In lateral projections, the posterior cruciate ligament is well extended when pressure is exerted on the tibia. The angle between the posterior cruciate ligament (thickness: 6–8 mm) and the tibial plateau is about 60°. The insertion of the posterior cruciate ligament is found 15–20 mm above the intercondylar eminence. The posterior contour is visible from the site of insertion to the superior margin of the medial meniscus because the large recess of the joint capsule (localized posterior to the medial femoral condyle) determines the posterior delimitation. Below this level, the posterior contour is not visible.

The anterior contour of the posterior cruciate ligament is as a rule only visible over a distance of a few millimeters at the

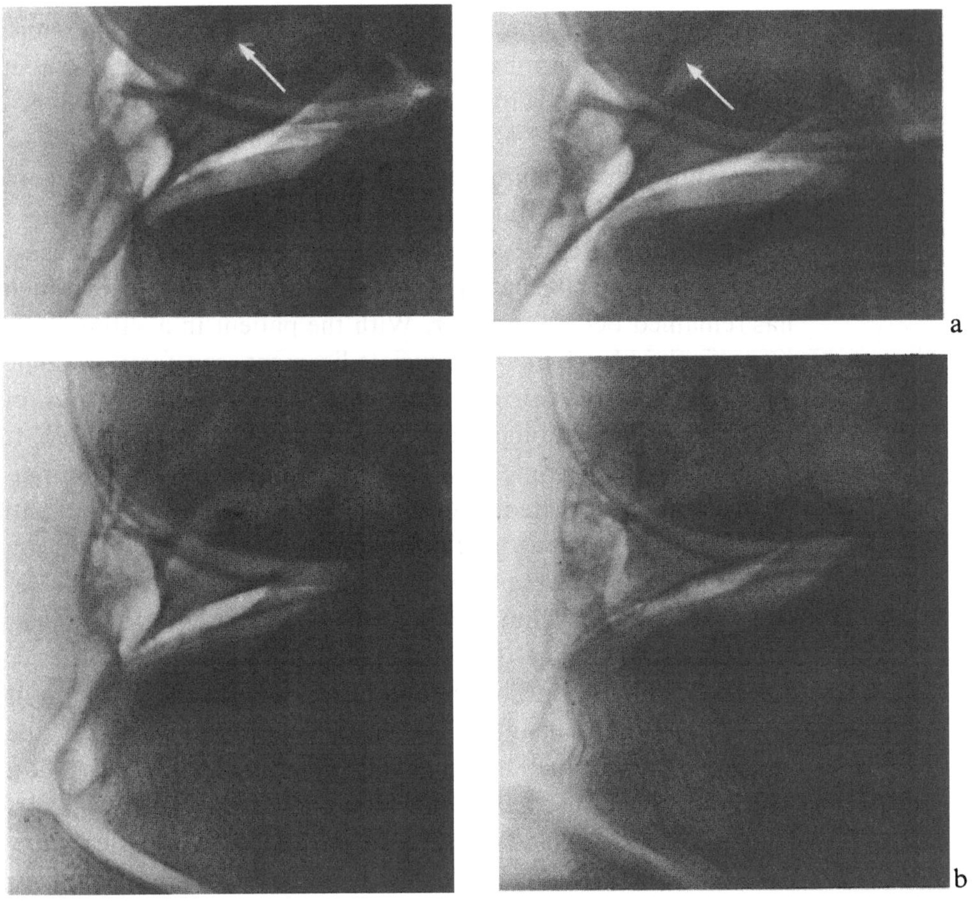

Fig. 134a and b. Two patients. Both pairs of stereoscopic photographs show the course of the popliteal tendon in detail projections of the lateral posterior horn. (a) Site of insertion of the popliteal tendon on the lateral aspect of the lateral condyle (*arrows*)

level of the medial part of the intercondylar eminence (Fig. 125). Of course the distance over which the anterior contour is visible depends on the degree of plication of the synovial membrane between the cruciate ligaments (Figs. 127, 129, 130, and 133).
The tendon of the popliteal muscle can be visible in the lateral projection as a band-like shadow of a few millimeters' width in the posterior compartment of the joint. The angle between the tendon and the tibial plateau is about 45°. On aimed arthrograms of the lateral posterior horn, the tendon of the popliteal muscle is regularly visible and can be followed as far as the site of insertion on the lateral aspect of the lateral femoral condyle. This site is about 1.5 cm above the femoral articular surface (Fig. 134a and b). In the lateral projection the tendon is less

readily distinguishable due to superposition on posterior cruciate ligament structures. As compared with the course of the posterior cruciate ligament, the tendon of the popliteal muscle takes a slightly flatter course, virtually parallel to the posterior margin of the intercondylar eminence (Fig. 138a). According to Lindblom (1938) the inferior delimitation is clearly defined at single contrast arthrography, and the superior delimitation is visible above the level of the lateral meniscus.

5.4 Etiology of Cruciate Ligament Ruptures

The nature of cruciate ligament lesions depends on the way in which and the site at which a trauma affects the knee joint. Luxation of the knee joint invariably causes cruciate ligament ruptures. A rupture of collateral ligaments frequently is associated with cruciate ligament lesions. Isolated cruciate ligament ruptures (usually of the anterior cruciate ligament) are rare. Anterior cruciate ligament rupture is often associated with rupture of the medial collateral ligament, and this combination leads to anteromedial instability. A combination of posterior cruciate ligament rupture with lateral collateral ligament rupture leads to posterolateral instability. At maximum extension of the knee joint, the anterior cruciate ligament is maximally tautened. A traumatic influence on the anterior aspect of the knee joint in this position leads to rupture of the anterior cruciate ligament and the posterior joint capsule.

A traumatic influence on the upper part of the lower leg when the knee is in 90° flexion leads to rupture of the posterior cruciate ligament (Baumgartl, 1964).

A cruciate ligament lesion can consist of hyperextension, partial rupture, or total rupture. When a bone fragment is detached from the tibia, the cruciate ligament itself can remain entirely intact (Fig. 135). Rupture at the femoral insertion of the cruciate ligaments usually does not involve avulsion of a bone fragment. Apart from these ruptures at the sites of insertion of the cruciate ligaments, ruptures of the midportion of these ligaments are found.

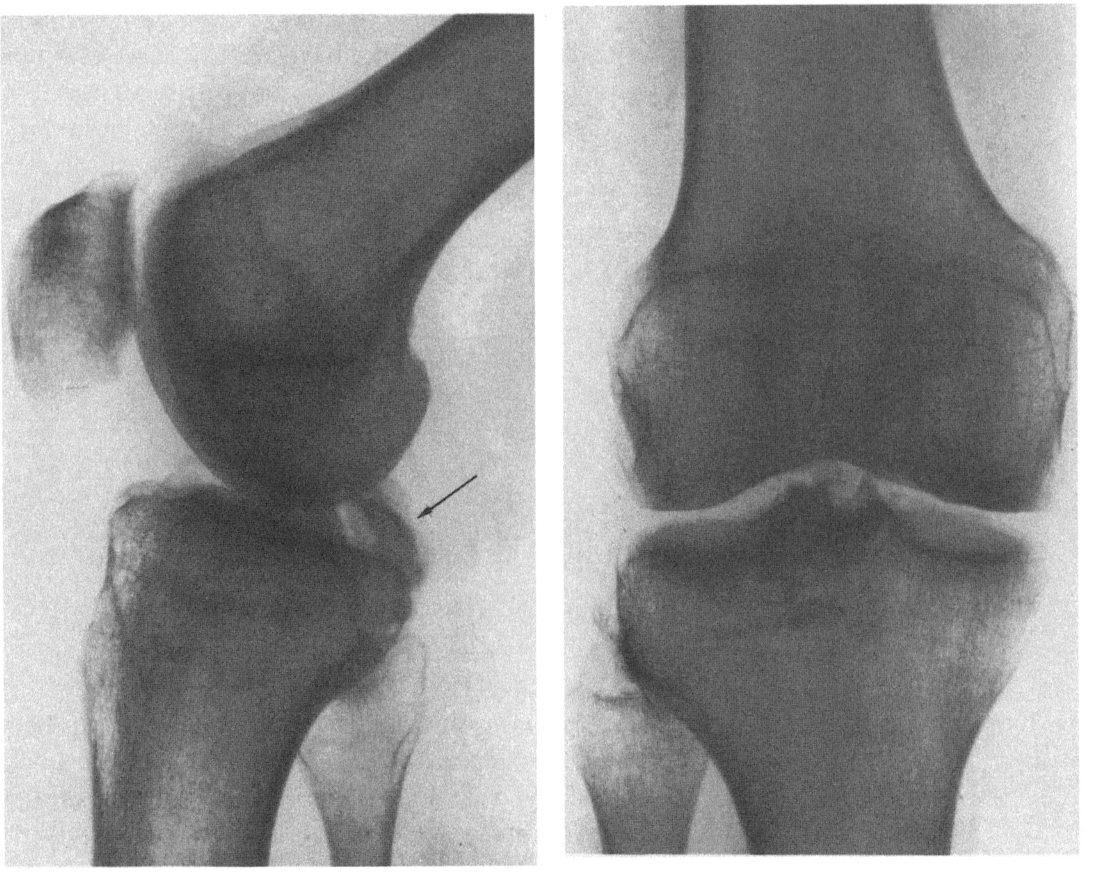

Fig. 135. Rupture of posterior cruciate ligament. Detached bone fragment of the tibial plateau visible (*arrow*). Arthroscopy: posterior cruciate ligament detached, but otherwise intact

5.5 Cruciate Ligament Pathology

A traumatic injury of the knee joint can lead to rupture of one or both cruciate ligaments, sometimes associated with ruptures of the menisci, the collateral ligaments, or the capsule. In some cases the injury tears away the cruciate ligament together with its insertion on the tibial plateau. Such lesions are readily diagnosed from radiographs without contrast medium (Fig. 135), but confusion with an osseous corpus liberum is of course possible. Arthrographically, cruciate ligament ruptures can lead to abnormal delimitation of the ligaments, abnormal displacement of the tibial plateau in relation to the femur, and irregular structures within the cruciate ligament compartments.

5.5.1 Abnormal Delimitation of the Cruciate Ligaments

An intact anterior cruciate ligament shows a sharp anterior delimitation in the lateral projection during stress (cf. Sect. 2.3). The cruciate ligament should be visible as a band-like radiolucency behind the sharp anterior delimitation. Total rupture of the anterior cruciate ligament causes disappearance of the sharp anterior delimitation. This need not only be visible in lateral projections; this symptom is also often present in detail projections of the anterior horn of the medial meniscus (Figs. 136, 137, and 145). After incomplete removal of intra-articular fluid, this (together with the contrast medium injected) can cause inconvenient superposition of the anterior cruciate ligament, as a result of which the anterior contour becomes invisible over a certain distance.

A normal depiction of the abrupt transition between cruciate ligament and femur is indicative of an intact anterior cruciate ligament (Figs. 126 and 138b). In the anterior compartment of the joint, the fluid level already mentioned can be projected at the site of the anterior cruciate ligament, thus imitating a sharp anterior delimitation of the ligament (Fig. 139). In these cases, however, the normal band-like radiolucency which denotes the normal anterior cruciate ligament is not observed behind the sharp line of demarcation between the two contrast media. If in addition the site of insertion of the anterior cruciate ligament on the femur cannot be identified, then the findings suggest the presence of an anterior cruciate ligament rupture (Fig. 139). Such a rupture does not imply that the synovial membrane is likewise ruptured. The latter may remain more or less intact. Particularly in the case of partial ligament rupture, rupture of the synovial membrane need not be total. In such cases arthrography may show an undulating contour of the anterior cruciate ligament, caused by partial cruciate ligament rupture, synovial reaction, or sometimes, blood clots.

After rupture of the posterior cruciate ligament the sharp posterior delimitation disappears. Given an intact anterior cruciate ligament, arthroscopic diagnosis of lesions of the posterior cruciate ligament is usually difficult. This enhances the importance of correct arthrographic diagnosis (Fig. 140).

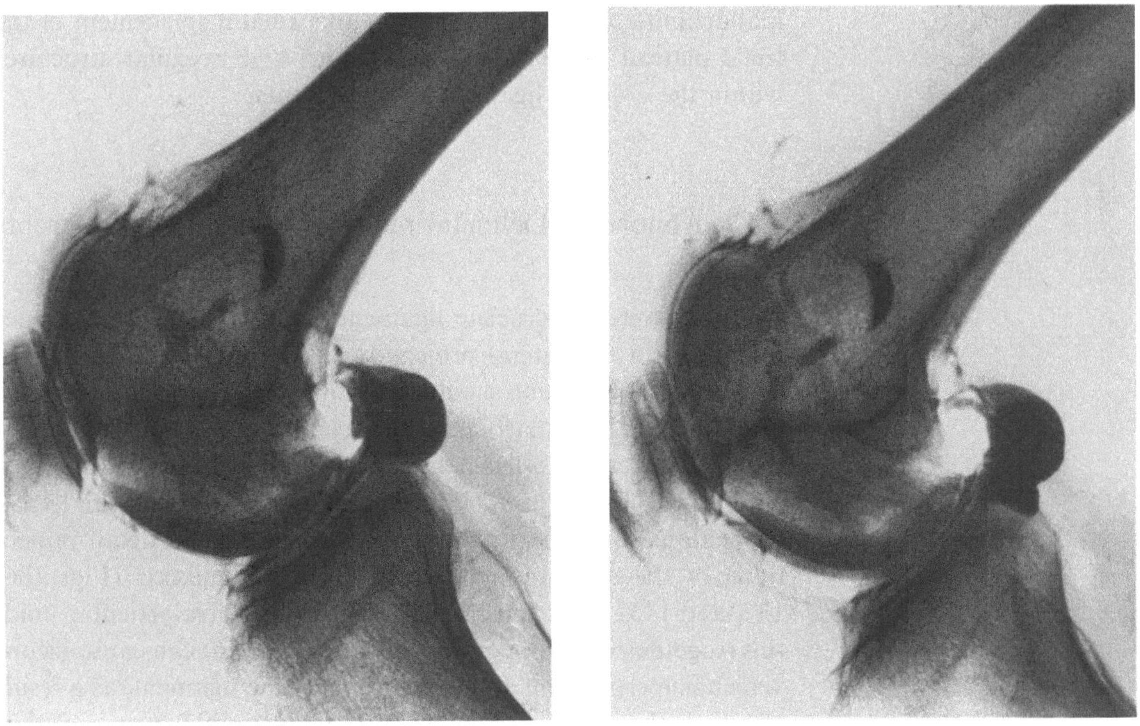

Fig. 136. Rupture of the anterior cruciate ligament. The normally sharp, rectilinear anterior delimitation is absent

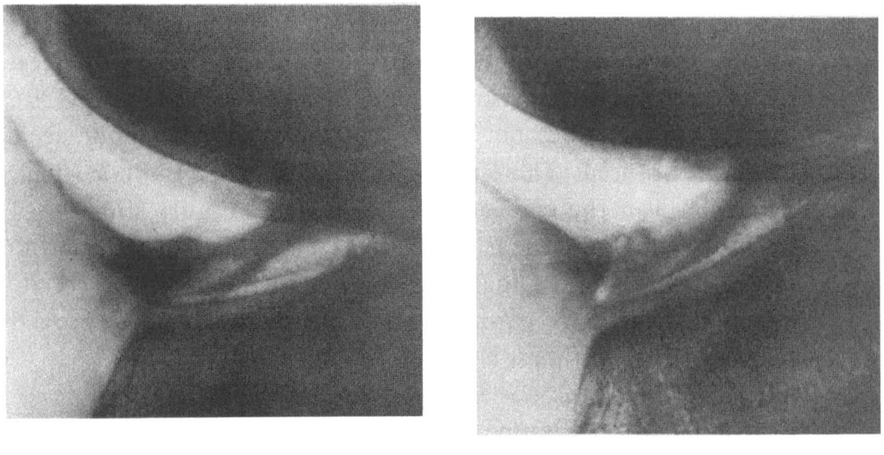

Fig. 137. Arthrographic diagnosis: rupture of the anterior horn of the medial meniscus. Arthroscopic diagnosis: rupture of the anterior cruciate ligament; meniscus intact. Conclusion: false positive arthrographic diagnosis of meniscal lesion

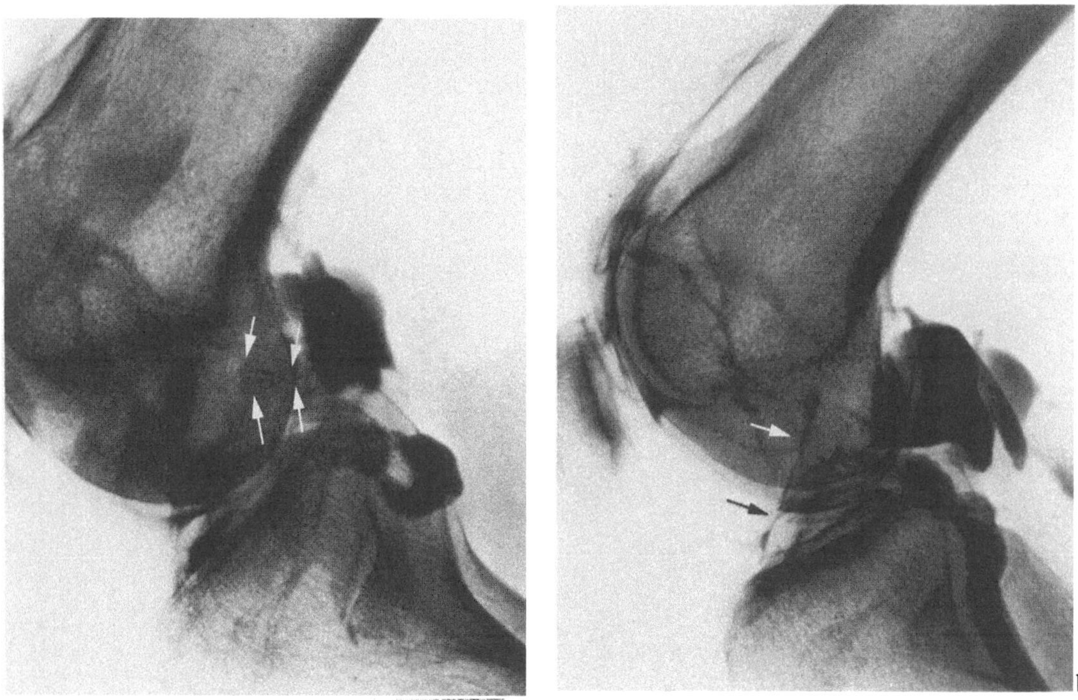

a b

Fig. 138. (a) Normal delimitation of the posterior cruciate ligament (*arrows*↓). Popliteal tendon visible (*arrows*↑). (b) Normal delimitation of the anterior cruciate ligament (*arrows*) and visible transition to intercondylar fossa. Low patella

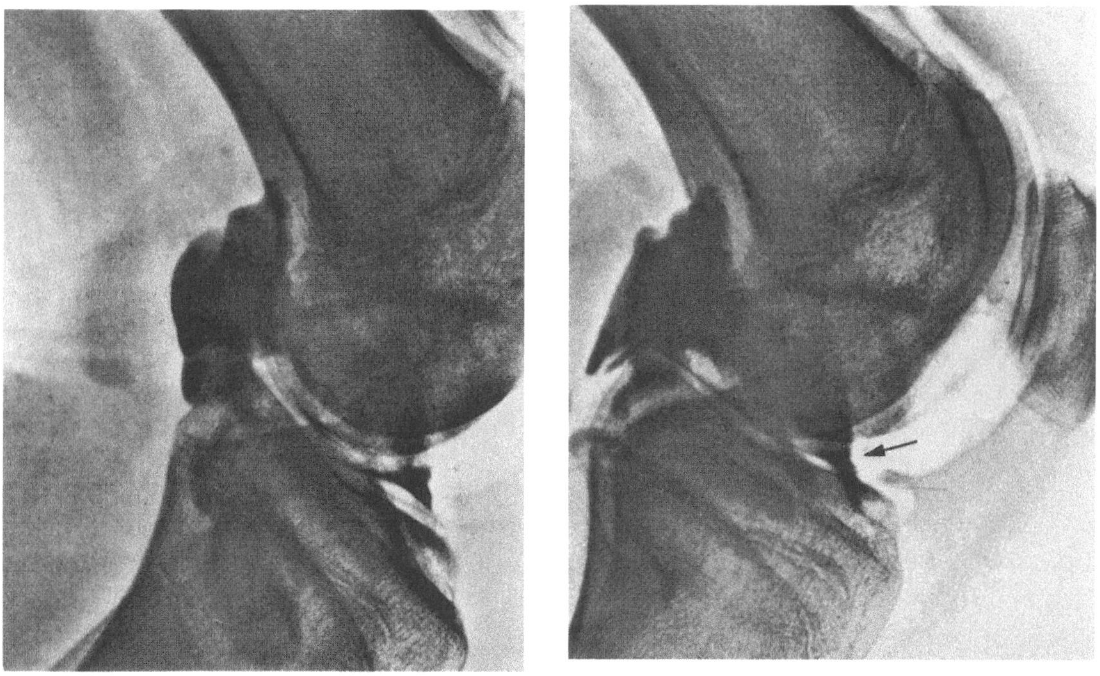

Fig. 139. Arthrographic diagnosis: intact anterior cruciate ligament. Arthroscopic diagnosis: ruptured anterior cruciate ligament. Conclusion: false negative arthrographic diagnosis. Explanation: the fluid level in the anterior compartment of the joint (*arrow*), imitated a sharp anterior delimitation of the anterior cruciate ligament

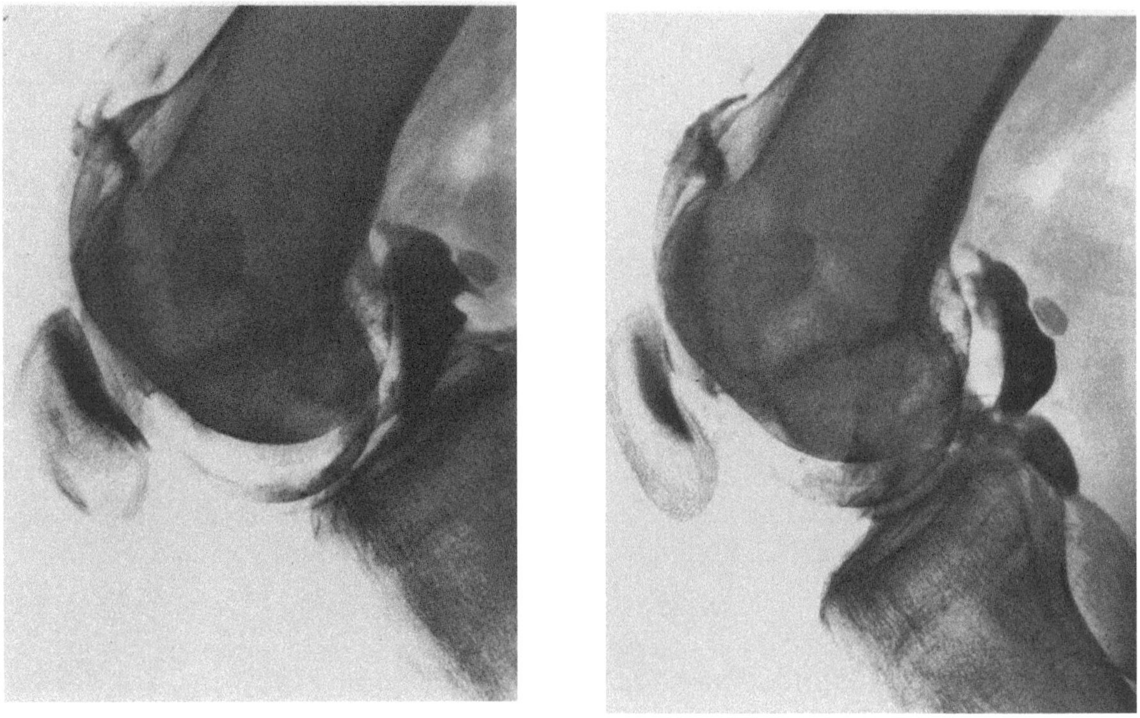

Fig. 140. Rupture of the posterior cruciate ligament. Marked displacement of the tibial plateau in dorsal direction

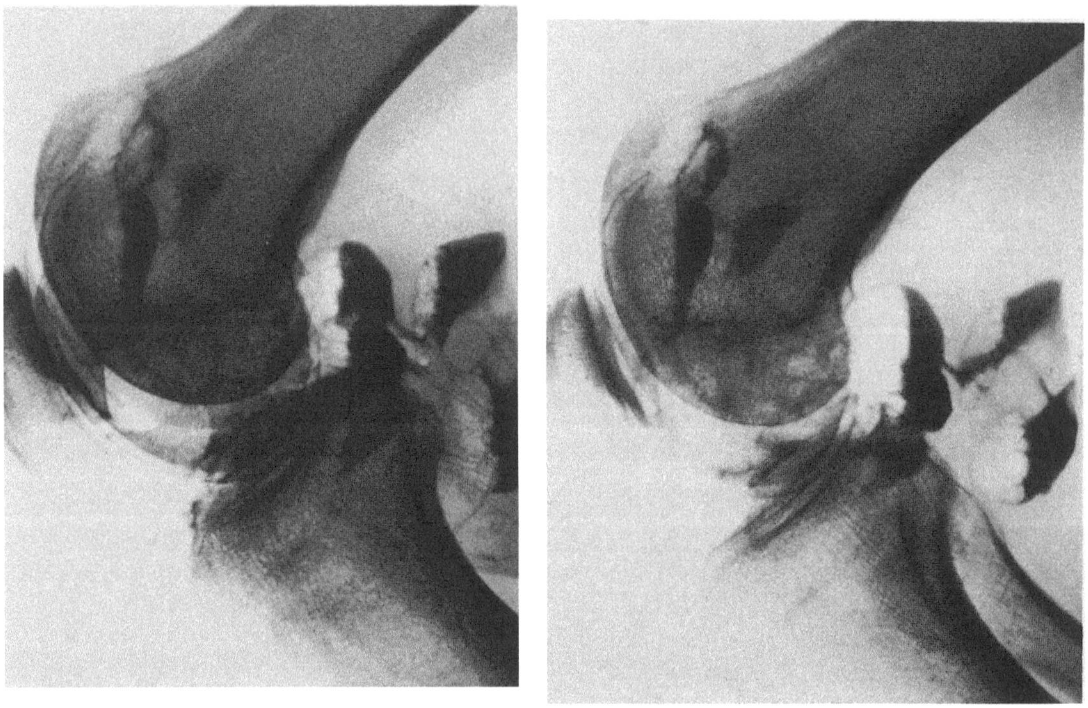

Fig. 141. Rupture of the anterior cruciate ligament. Conspicuously increased distance between femoral condyles and anterior aspect of tibial plateau. No anterior delimitation of the anterior cruciate ligament. Large semimembranosogastrocnemial bursa

5.5.2 Abnormal Displacement of the Tibia in Relation to the Femur

The two lateral projections of the knee joint, during stress on the anterior and the posterior cruciate ligament, respectively, normally show a tibiofemoral displacement of no more than 5–10 mm (Figs. 126 and 127). This displacement is largely dependent on the patient's ability to relax the knee. Moreover, exact measurement of the displacement is impeded when lower leg rotation is not the same in the two projections. It should be noted that this rotation can be easily verified from the position of the head of the fibula. Flaccidity of the collateral ligaments as a rule increases rotation.

After rupture of the anterior cruciate ligament, the projection in 90° flexion and during stress often reveals a conspicuous increase in the distance between the femoral condyles and the anterior aspect of the tibial plateau. This is usually more evident than the ventral displacement of the tibial plateau in relation to the femoral condyles (Figs. 141 and 142). The latter displacement, clinically known as drawer sign (*vordere Schublade*), is usually not much more than 10 mm, probably due to the stabilizing influence of the normal posterior cruciate ligament when the knee is flexed 90°.

After a lesion of the posterior cruciate ligament, the dorsal displacement of the tibia (*hintere Schublade*) is generally much more pronounced. In our series of patients the displacement after posterior cruciate ligament ruptures ranged from 15 to 30 mm (Figs. 140, 143, and 144).

Figs. 142–145 see page 114 and 115.

Fig. 142. Rupture of the anterior cruciate ligament. Enlarged distance between femoral condyles and anterior aspect of tibial plateau. No anterior delimitation of cruciate ligament

Fig. 143. Rupture of the posterior cruciate ligament. Marked dorsal displacement of the tibial plateau

Fig. 144. Rupture of the posterior cruciate ligament. Marked dorsal displacement of the tibial plateau

Fig. 145. Rupture of both cruciate ligaments. No anterior delimitation of anterior cruciate ligament. Marked ventral and dorsal displacement of the tibial plateau

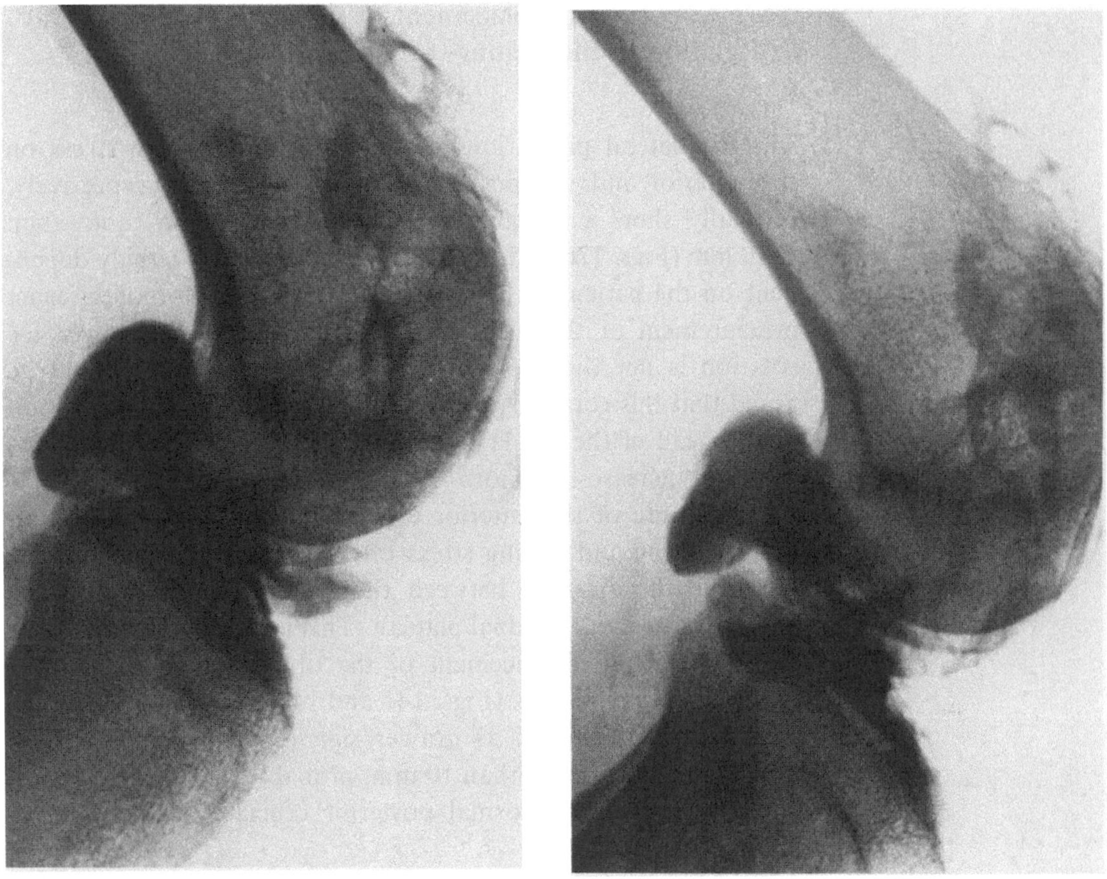

Fig. 142

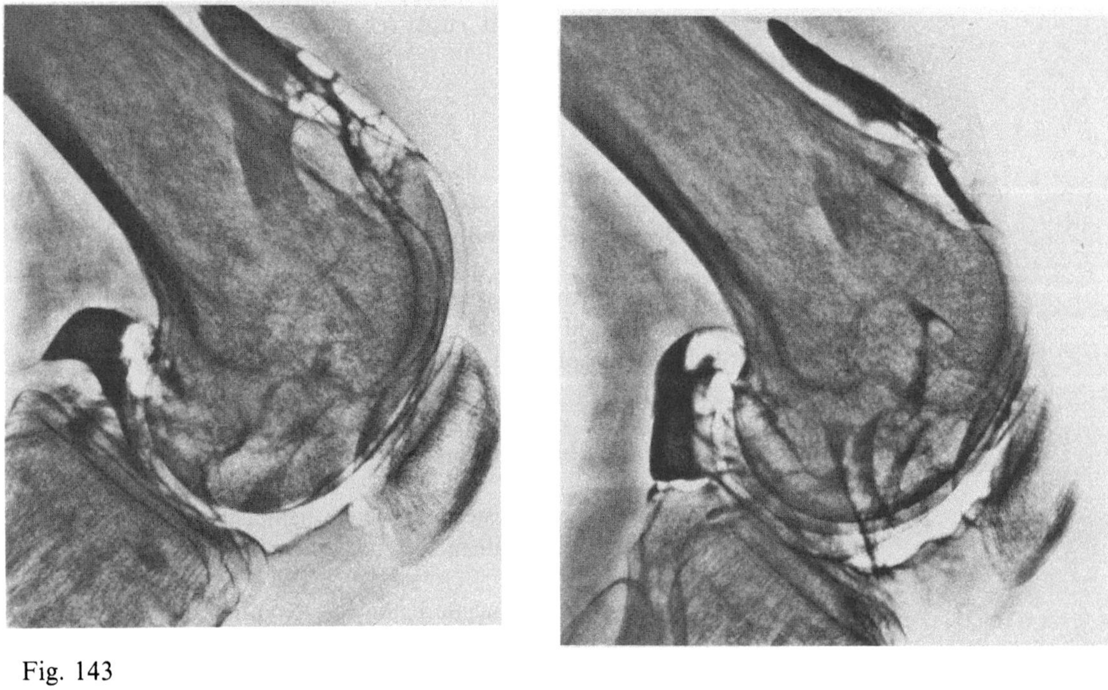

Fig. 143

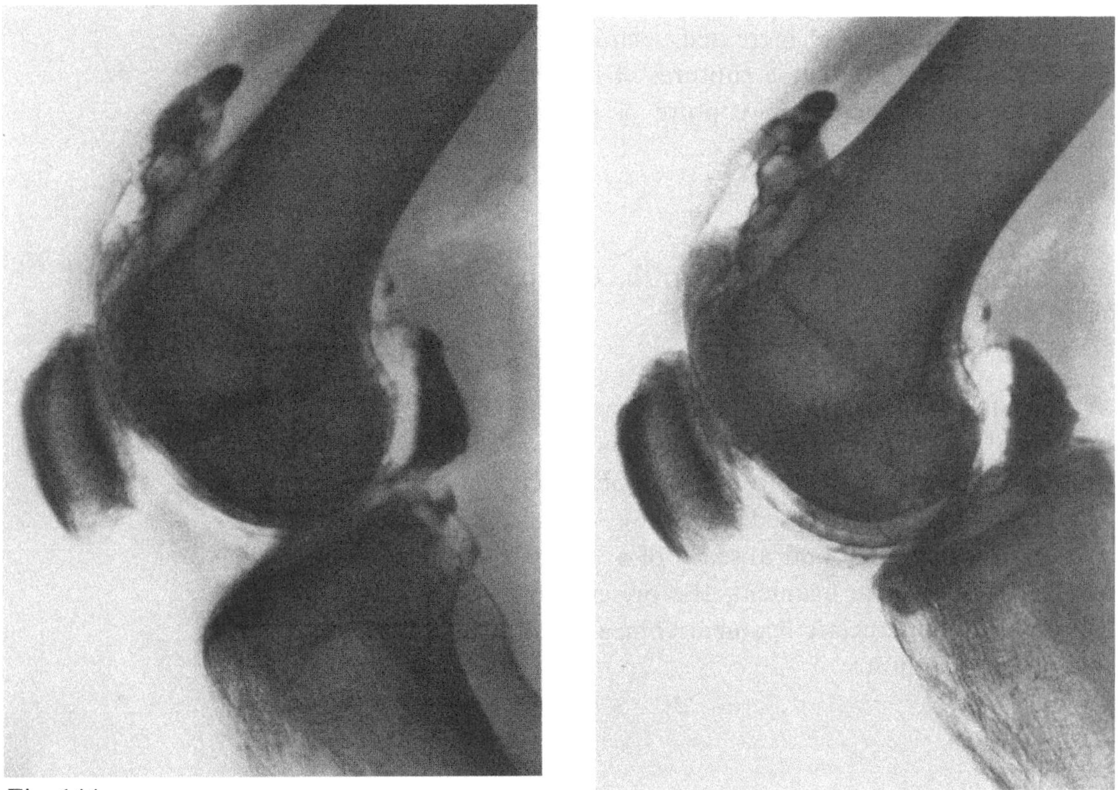

Fig. 144

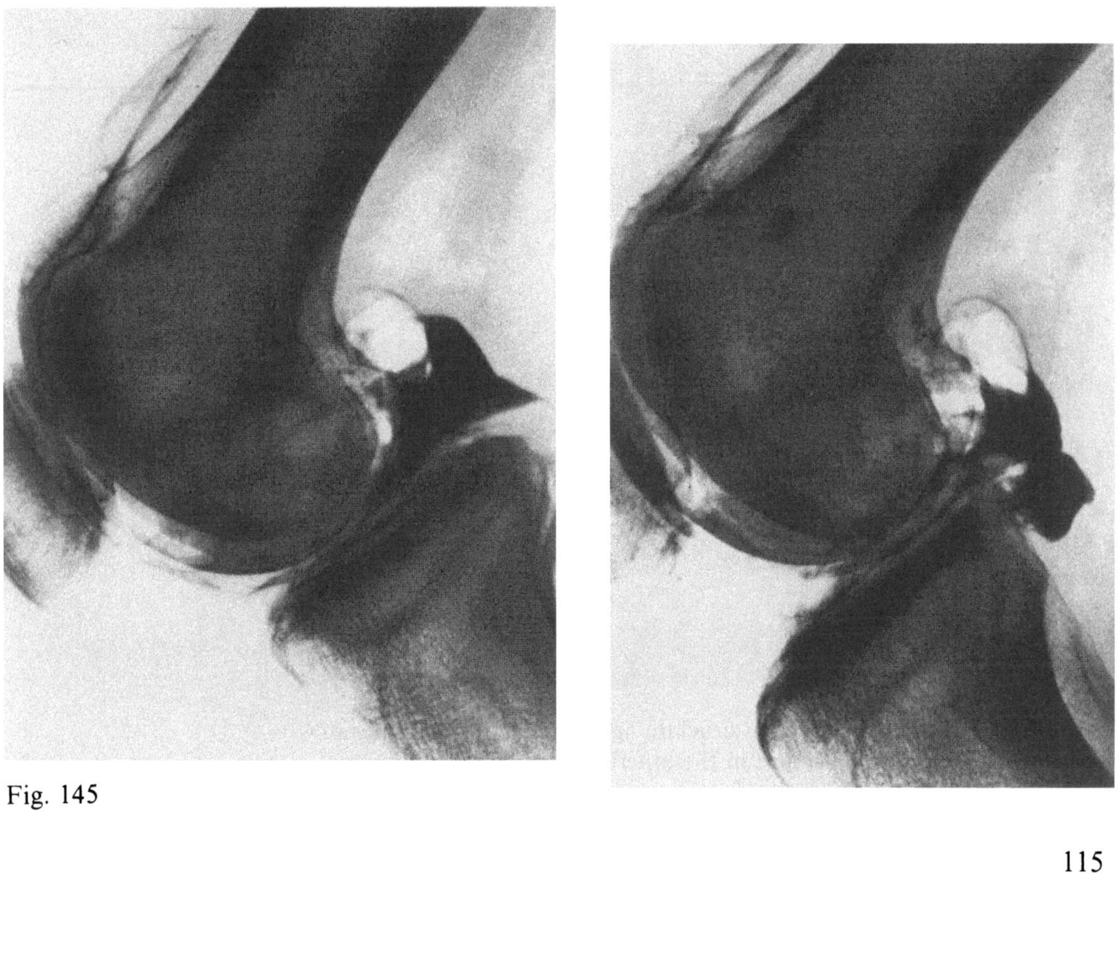

Fig. 145

After rupture of both the anterior and the posterior cruciate ligaments, there may be increased ventral as well as dorsal displacement (Fig. 145). These ruptures of both cruciate ligaments are always associated with rupture of one or both collateral ligaments and meniscal lesions.

5.5.3 Irregular Structures Within the Cruciate Ligament Compartments

At the site where a normal cruciate ligament should be present, abnormal arthrographic shadows may be observed after a rupture. It is often impossible to establish on which anatomic structures these shadows are based (Fig. 146). Apart from the presence of abnormal mobility and absence of a distinct delimitation of the anterior cruciate ligament, the presence of these abnormal structures in the cruciate ligament compartment is an additional indication of rupture.

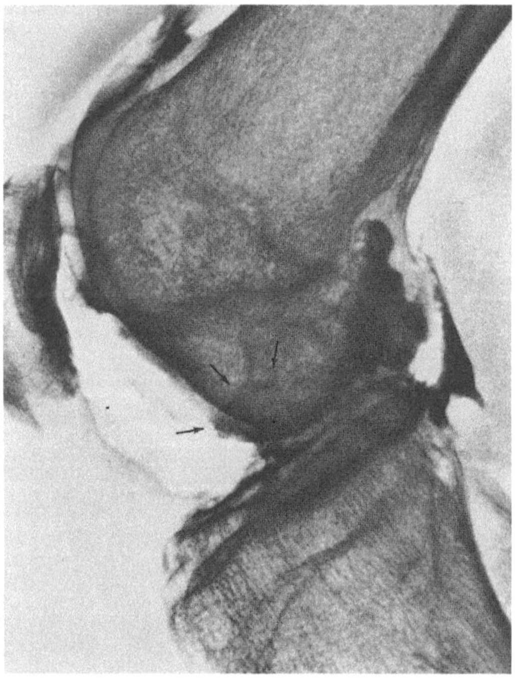

Fig. 146. Rupture of the anterior cruciate ligament. No sharp anterior delimitation. Irregular structure in the anterior cruciate ligament compartment (*arrows*)

5.6 Accuracy of Arthrographic Cruciate Ligament Diagnosis

According to Liljedahl et al. (1966), single contrast arthrography (combined with tomography if necessary) is the method of choice in demonstrating cruciate ligament lesions. They reported an accuracy of about 90%. Nicholas et al. (1970), using double contrast arthrography, achieved a good correlation with clinical and operative findings in about 50% of their patients.

As already mentioned in the discussion of the accuracy of double contrast arthrography in diagnosing meniscal lesions, comparison of accuracy rates between arthrography and surgery on the one hand, and arthrography and arthroscopy on the other, is biased by the fact that an operation is often not performed on patients whose clinical and arthrographic findings are not indicative of a cruciate ligament lesion. In such cases an erroneous arthrographic diagnosis is not verified.

The correlation between arthrographic and arthroscopic diagnosis was determined in 122 consecutive patients in our series. Of the 92 patients in whom arthrography failed to reveal any cruciate ligament lesion, 84 (91%) showed a positive correlation with arthroscopic findings (Table 9). In the remaining 8 patients arthrography was false negative. Cruciate ligament rupture was correctly diagnosed arthrographically in 24 of 30 patients (80%), while a false positive result was obtained in 6 patients (20%).

Table 9. Correlation between double contrast arthrography and arthroscopy in ruptures of the cruciate ligaments in patients in whom arthrography led to the diagnoses "no lesions" and "ruptured cruciate ligament"

Arthrography	Pos. correlation arthrography – arthroscopy	False neg. arthrogram	False pos. arthrogram	Number of patients
No abnormalities	84 (91%)	8 (9%)	–	92
Cruciate ligament rupture	24 (80%)	–	6 (20%)	30
				122

Disregarding the arthrographic diagnosis "no lesion" in the table and taking the arthroscopic diagnosis "cruciate ligament rupture" as a starting-point, the accuracy of arthrographic diagnosis is found to be significantly lower (Table 10).

Table 10. Correlation between double contrast arthrography and arthroscopy in 122 patients; cruciate ligament ruptures were diagnosed in 32. The arthrographic diagnosis was false positive in 6 patients and false negative in 8. The anterior cruciate ligament was ruptured in 26 and the posterior cruciate ligament in 6 cases

Arthrography	Arthroscopy	Anterior	Posterior	Normal
Correct +	Correct +	18	4	84
Correct +	Dubious	–	2	
False +	Correct –	(6)	–	
False –	Correct +	8	–	
Number of lesions		26 (6)	6	

In the arthrographic diagnosis of anterior cruciate ligament ruptures, absence of the anterior delimitation is the most reliable symptom. In double contrast arthrography of posterior cruciate ligament ruptures, anteroposterior displacement is of special importance. This proved to be present in the majority of cases.

6 Joint Capsule, Collateral Ligaments, Hoffa Body, and Bursae

This chapter discusses the anatomy and the radiodiagnostically important pathology of the interrelated structures of capsule, collateral ligaments, Hoffa body, and bursae.

6.1 Capsule, Hoffa Body, and Collateral Ligaments

The outer part of the joint capsule consists of a firm fibrous membrane which, on the inside, is lined with synovial membrane. On the anterior side of the femur the capsule is attached to the bone about 2 cm above the femoral cartilage. The distance between capsule insertion and cartilage surface on the posterior side is 1 cm. On the anterior side of the femur the capsule forms an ample suprapatellar bursa, which permits the normal mobility of the joint. The capsule localized behind the quadriceps tendon and patellar retinacula envelops the patella and finally inserts on the anterior aspect of the tibia. The synovial membrane is separated from the fibrous capsule by a thin layer of adipose tissue in which blood vessels, nerves, and low-density connective tissue are localized. Beside the patella, a few fairly flat adipose folds, lined with synovial membrane, ensure adequate adaptation between capsule and femoral condyles (Fig. 147). The synovial membrane lines the alar folds of the Hoffa body below the patella. A long fold of the synovial membrane, which largely contains adipose tissue, connects the Hoffa body to the intercondylar fossa (Fig. 132). The Hoffa body extends from the inferior aspect of the patella to the anterosuperior aspect of the tibia, thus filling the space between capsule, patella, femoral condyles, anterior cruciate ligament and menisci. The Hoffa body is clearly visible on soft-tissue radiographs (Fig. 148). In some individuals the Hoffa body is very large, so that the anterior horn area of the meniscus is entirely or almost entirely covered, and the central part of the meniscus is only just visible ventral to the large Hoffa body (Fig. 149; also Fig. 14). A mobile fold of the

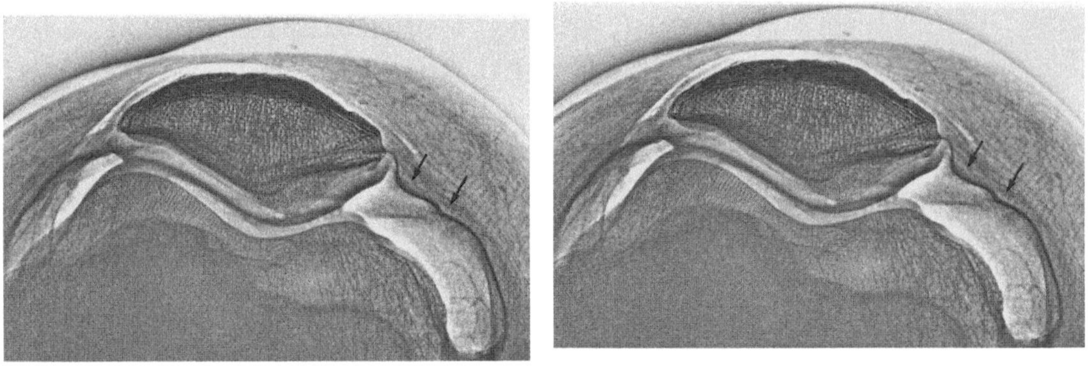

Fig. 147. Xerography of patellofemoral joint. Relatively flat folds lined with synovial tissue ensure adequate adaptation between capsule and femoral condyles (*arrows*)

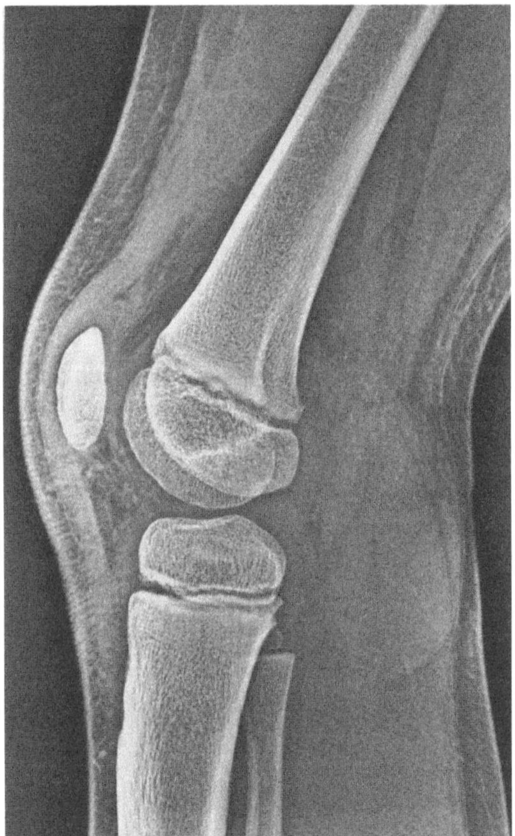

Fig. 148. Xerography of knee joint, clearly showing soft tissues such as the Hoffa body. Large oval-shaped soft-tissue shadow on the posterior side of the joint. Clinical features: "Baker cyst"

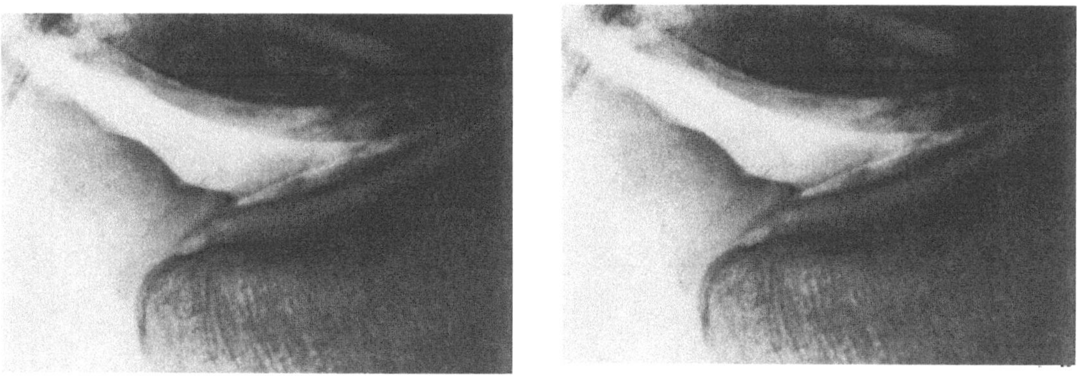

a b

Fig. 149. (a) Large Hoffa body covering a large part of the meniscus; however, the central part of the medial meniscus remains visible (b)

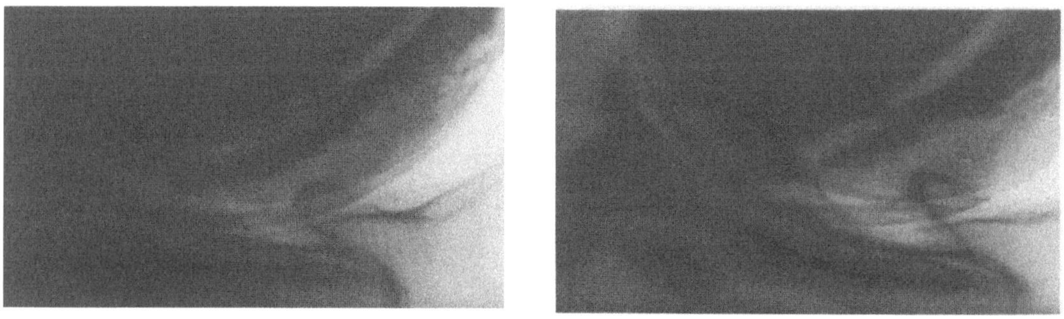

a

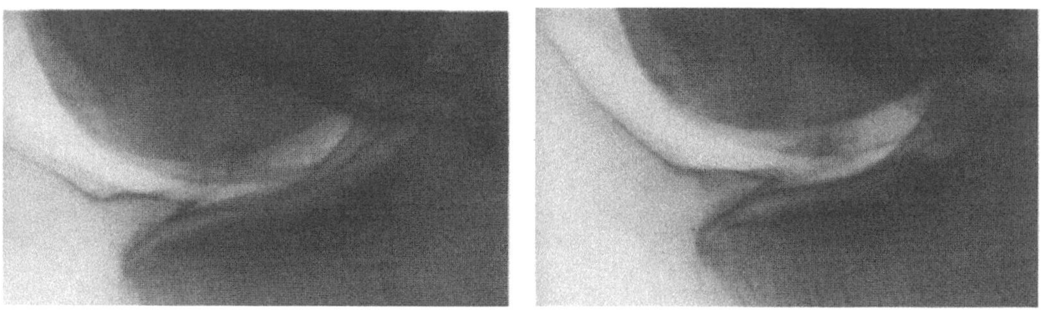

b

Fig. 150a–c. Female, age 18. (a) Details projections of anterior horn with Hoffa flake. (b) Examination one year later: situation unchanged. (c) see page 143

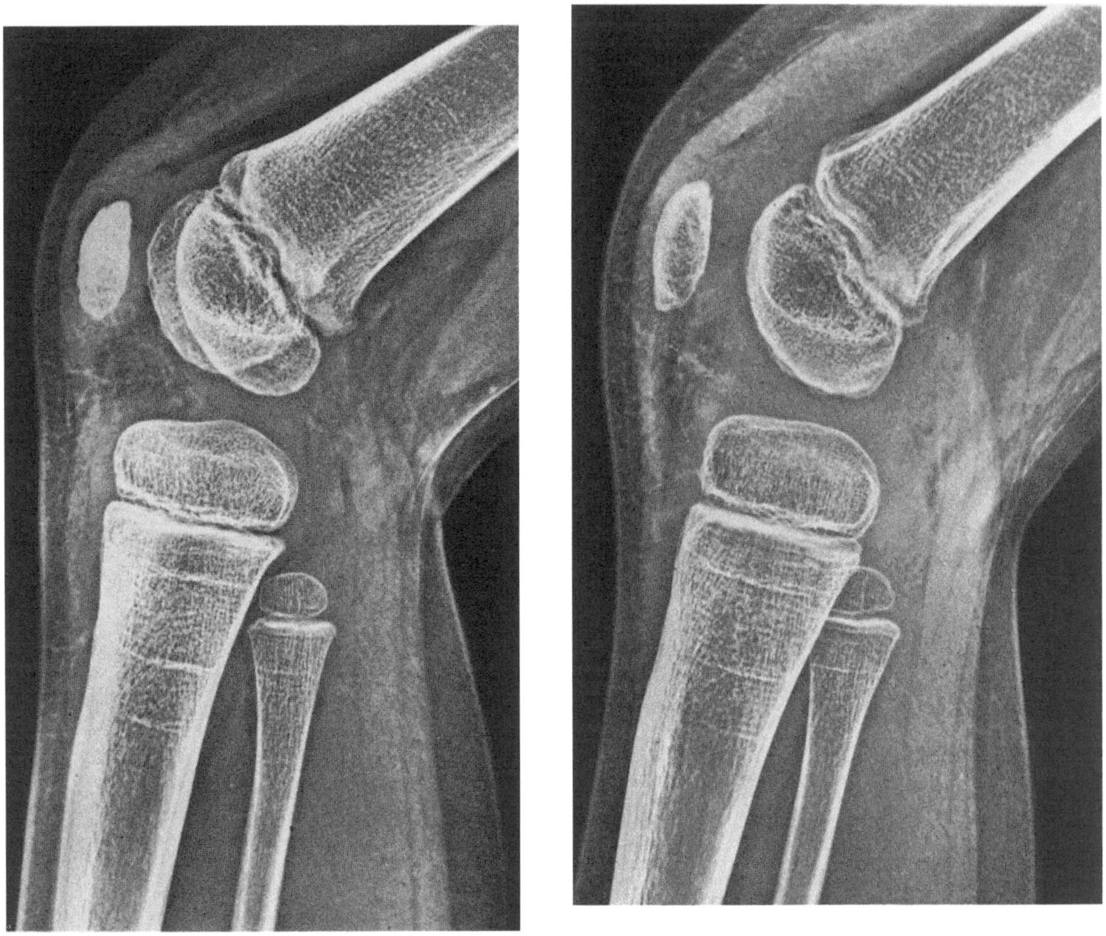

Fig. 151. Xerography of both knees. Right: unmistakable changes in the depiction of soft tissues as a result of chronic synovitis

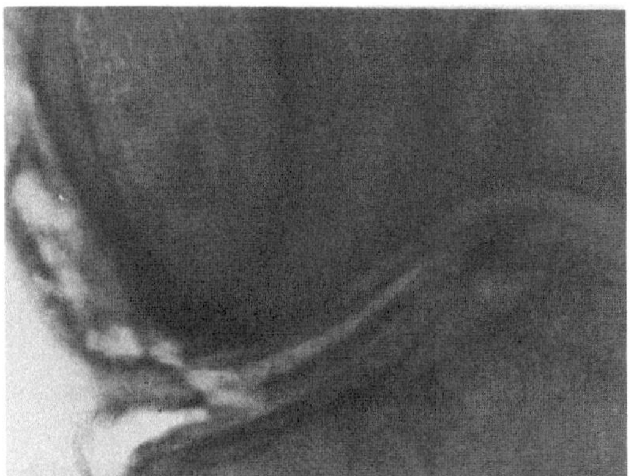

Fig. 152. Rheumatoid arthritis. Marked synovitis and narrowing of articular cartilage. Secondary degeneration of meniscal cartilage

adipose tissue in the area of the medial anterior horn can imitate a meniscal lesion (Fig. 150).

The synovial membrane lines the two cruciate ligaments from the ventral side, as described in Chap. 5. This lining of the cruciate ligaments continues into the fibrous capsule on the posterior side. On the posterior side the joint capsule is thus divided into two compartments (Fig. 9). On both sides of the knee joint the capsule connects the femoral part just above the cartilage margin with the tibial part about 5 mm below the cartilage surface. The synovial membrane can be very easily inspected by arthroscopy. In virtually all intra-articular lesions the synovial membrane shows a pathologic appearance (Eikelaar, 1975). There is usually synovitis. In such cases the synovial villi show edema-

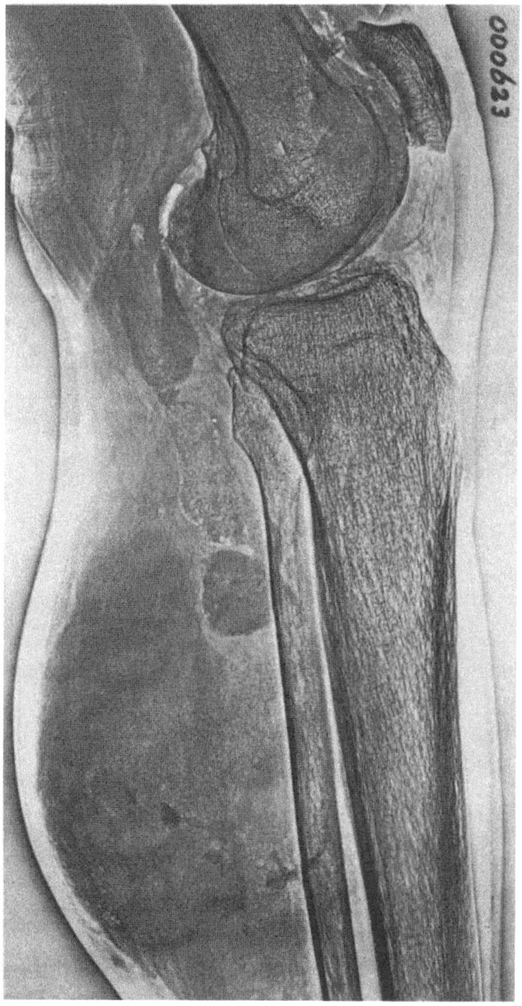

Fig. 153. Rheumatoid arthritis. Very large semimembranosogastrocnemial bursa extending deep into the calf. Clinical features: "Baker cyst"

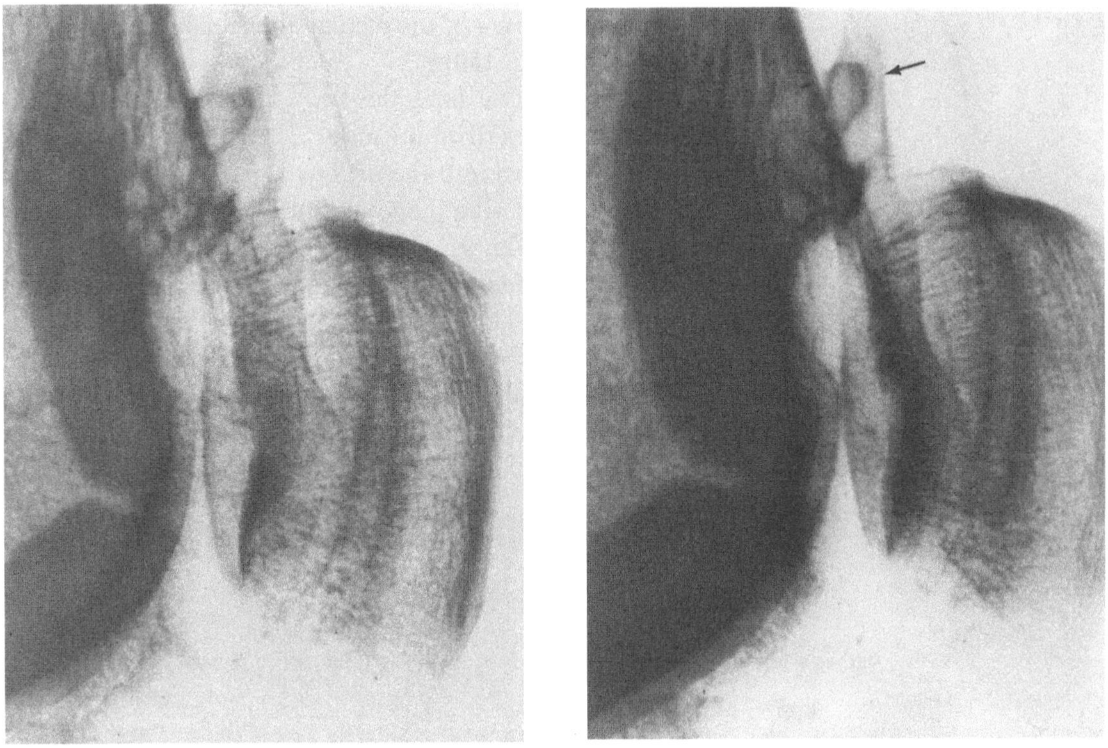

Fig. 154. Small polypous swelling in the suprapatellar bursa (*arrow*). Histology: features of chronic inflammation

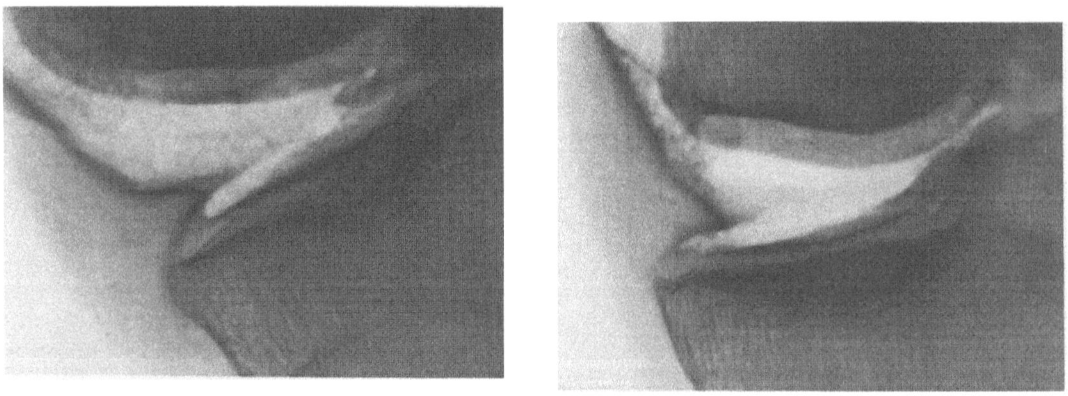

Fig. 155. Old rupture of medial collateral ligament. Marked dilatation of medial intra-articular space

tous swelling and hyperemia. These synovial changes are observed in inflammations (nonspecific, specific, and rheumatoid arthritis). Chronic irritation of the synovial membrane also exists in postoperative articular lesions. This irritation usually leads to chronic or recurrent hydrops (Fig. 151). In such cases the synovial membrane, which normally is sharply defined, shows blurred contours (Fig. 152). The entire synovial membrane is

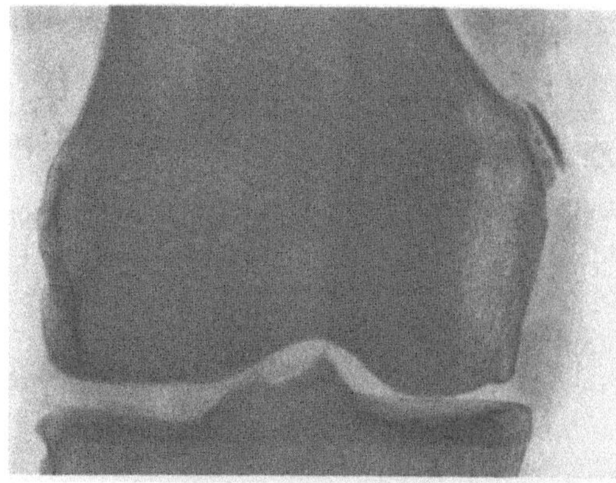

Fig. 156. Calcification named after Pelligrini Stieda. Old rupture of medial collateral ligament

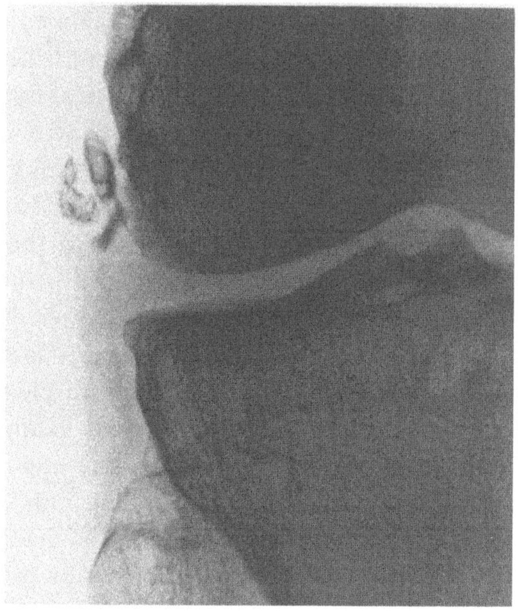

a

b

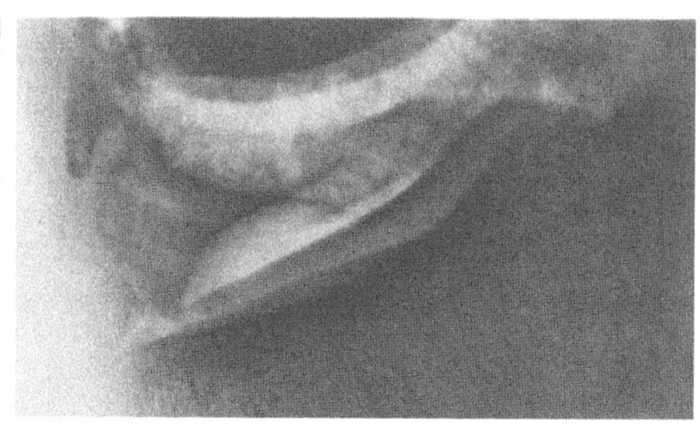

Fig. 157. (a) Old rupture of lateral collateral ligament. Calcifications beside the lateral femoral condyle. (b) Arthrography: marked dilatation of the lateral intra-articular space

involved in the process, and consequently, the Hoffa body and the cruciate ligaments are likewise irregularly delimited.

Particularly in rheumatoid arthritis the semimembranosogastrocnemial bursa is often greatly dilatated (Fig. 153). The synovial membrane is often markedly nodular in villinodular synovitis (Bessler et al., 1963). Solitary polypous swelling of the capsule is occasionally observed (Fig. 154). The features of capsular chondromatosis can be radiologically demonstrated in the same way. The subsequently calcified cartilaginous swellings of the synovial membrane can be clearly demonstrated by radiologic examination without contrast medium. Especially in the later stages of this abnormality, arthrography is of no significance.

On the medial side of the knee, the collateral ligament is firmly connected to the fibrous capsule and therefore also to the medial meniscus. The ligament can be divided into a superficial and a deep part. The superficial part of the ligament arises from the medial femoral epicondyle and inserts on the tibia 5–8 cm below the articular cavity. The deeper part arises from the medial femoral condyle and inserts on the tibia immediately below the articular cavity. This part of the ligament is firmly attached to the joint capsule. Rupture of the medial collateral ligament therefore often causes rupture of the fibrous capsule and the synovial membrane, thus giving rise to hemarthros. In such injuries the medial meniscus is also regularly ruptured because its base is firmly connected to the deeper part of the ligament. In addition, both menisci are attached to the tibia by the arcuate ligaments. A fresh rupture of the medial collateral ligament is indirectly demonstrable by arthrography in that contrast medium is observed outside the articular cavity. The capsular rupture closes after a few days. In such circumstances arthrographic examination after closure of the defect merely reveals that the medial articular cavity is readily dilatable, but no contrast medium outside the joint capsule is observed. An old rupture of the medial collateral ligament can be diagnosed in an anteroposterior projection on the basis of the calcification, which has been given the name of Pelligrini Stieda (Figs. 155 and 156).

The lateral collateral ligament connects the lateral femoral epicondyle to the head of the fibula. The ligament is pencil thick and attached to the joint capsule only by low-density connective tissue. Rupture of the lateral collateral ligament, too, is associated with dilatation of the lateral articular cavity. In older lesions calcifications may be visible at the site of insertion of the lateral ligament on the femur (Fig. 157).

6.2 Bursae

The articular cavity of the knee connects with several bursae. In this section these bursae are discussed in so far as they are of importance in arthrography.

6.2.1 Suprapatellar Bursa

The proximal recurvation fold of this bursa has only little attachment to adjacent parts, thus ensuring adequate mobility in flexion and extension of the knee. The bursa has an ample communication with the articular cavity, but in rare cases this communication is absent. This results from the failure of the fetal bursa below the quadriceps muscle to connect with the articular cavity.

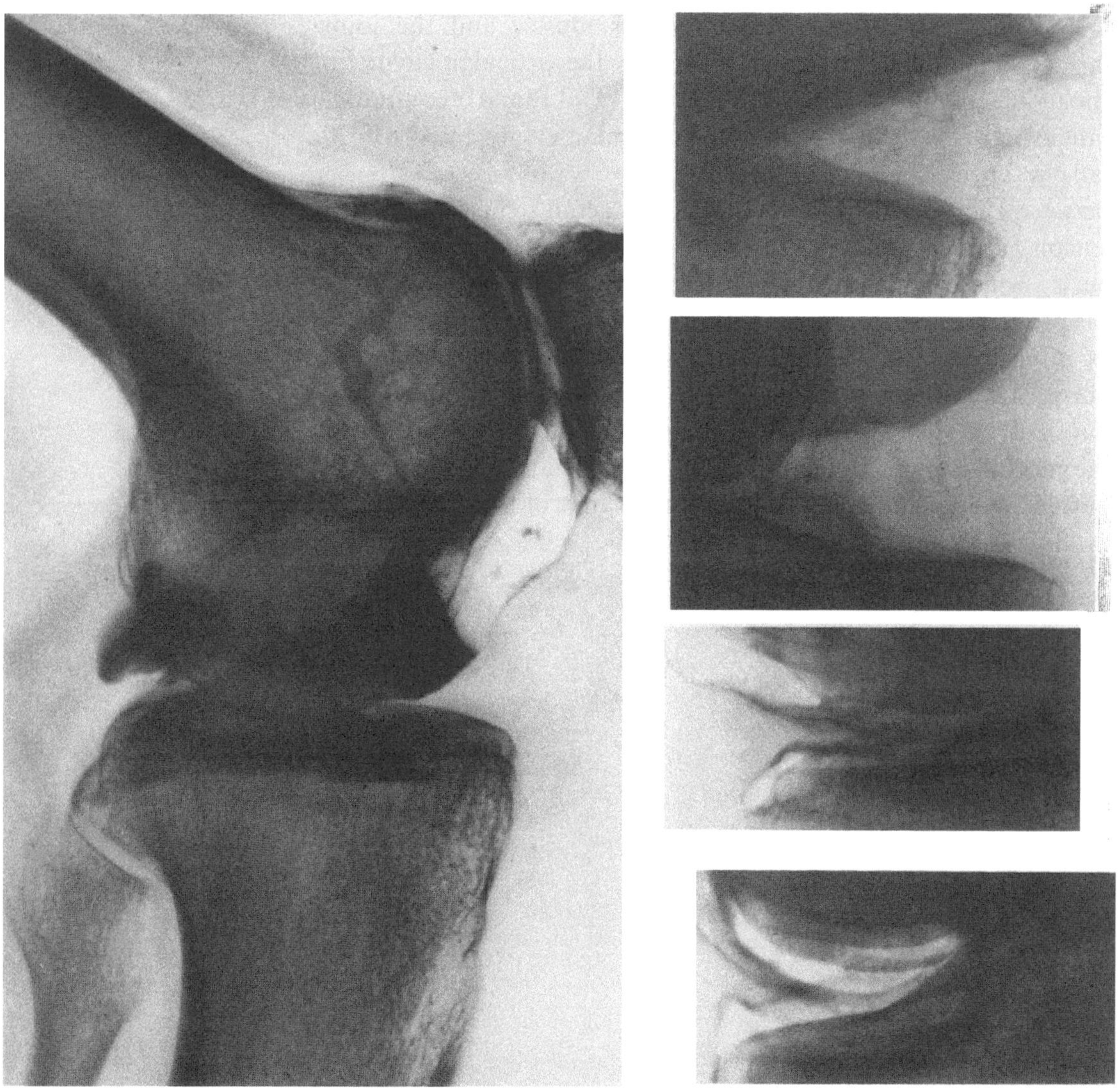

b

c

a

Fig. 158 a–c. Posttraumatic state. After lateral injection of contrast medium, only the lateral articular cavity fills (c). Separation between medial (b) and lateral compartment of the joint (arthroscopically confirmed). No filled suprapatellar bursa (a)

In some cases the articular cavity can post-traumatically be divided into two compartments separated by a septum. This is illustrated in Fig. 158; in this case it was found that contrast medium injected on the lateral side failed to enter the medial articular cavity and the suprapatellar bursa.

6.2.2 Semimembranosogastrocnemial Bursa

The medial head of the gastrocnemius muscle arises from the medial posterior aspect of the femur. The gastrocnemial bursa is localized between the tendon of this muscle and the joint capsule. This bursa communicates with the articular cavity in about 50% of individuals. Wilson et al. (1938) found a communication between the bursa and the articular cavity in 17 of 30 cadaver knees examined.

Between the medial head of the gastrocnemius muscle and the tendon of the semimembranosus muscle lies the semimembranous bursa, which in the majority of cases communicates with the gastrocnemial bursa. Most authors describe these two bursae as an entity which they call the semimembranosogastrocnemial bursa. The communication between gastrocnemial bursa and joint capsule is localized high in the posterior large recess around the medial femoral condyle (Figs. 159, 160, and 164). The two bursae are often indistinguishable, and in view of the interrelated-

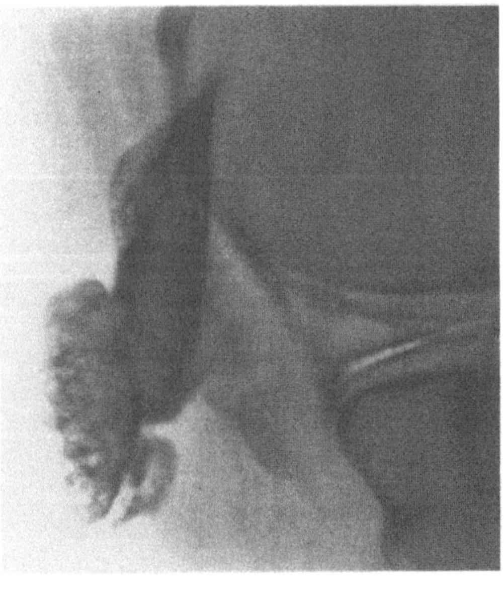

Fig. 159. Semimembranosogastrocnemial bursa

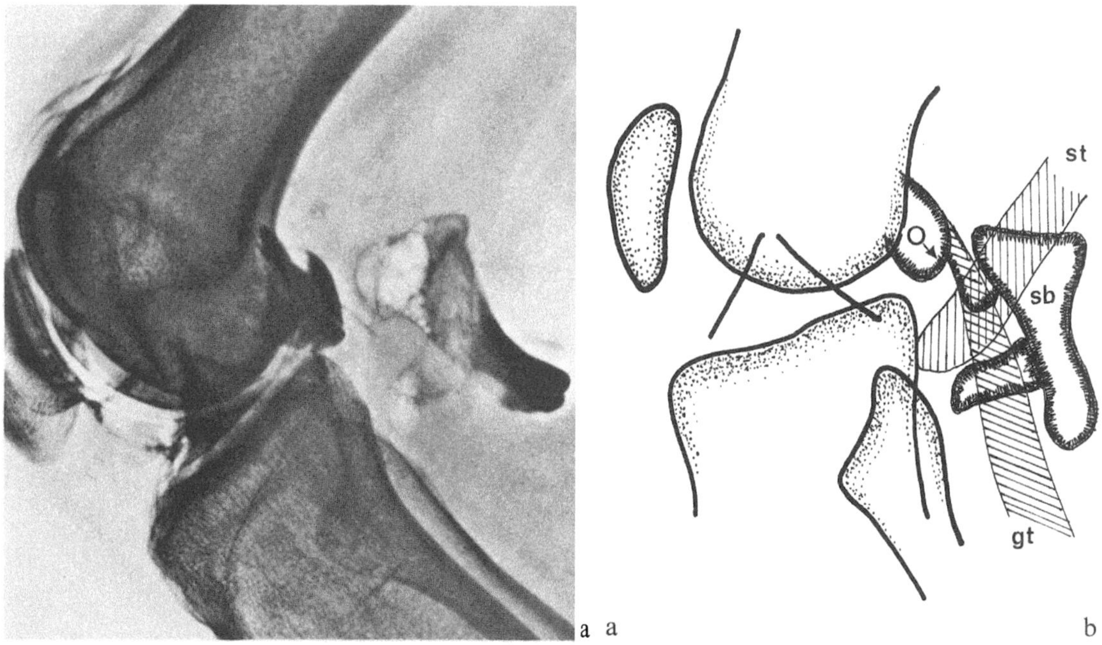

Fig. 160. (a) Radiograph; (b) drawing from (a). gt. gastrocnemius tendon; sb. semimembranosogastrocnemial bursa; st. semimembranosus tendon; O. Opening from the articular cavity to bursa

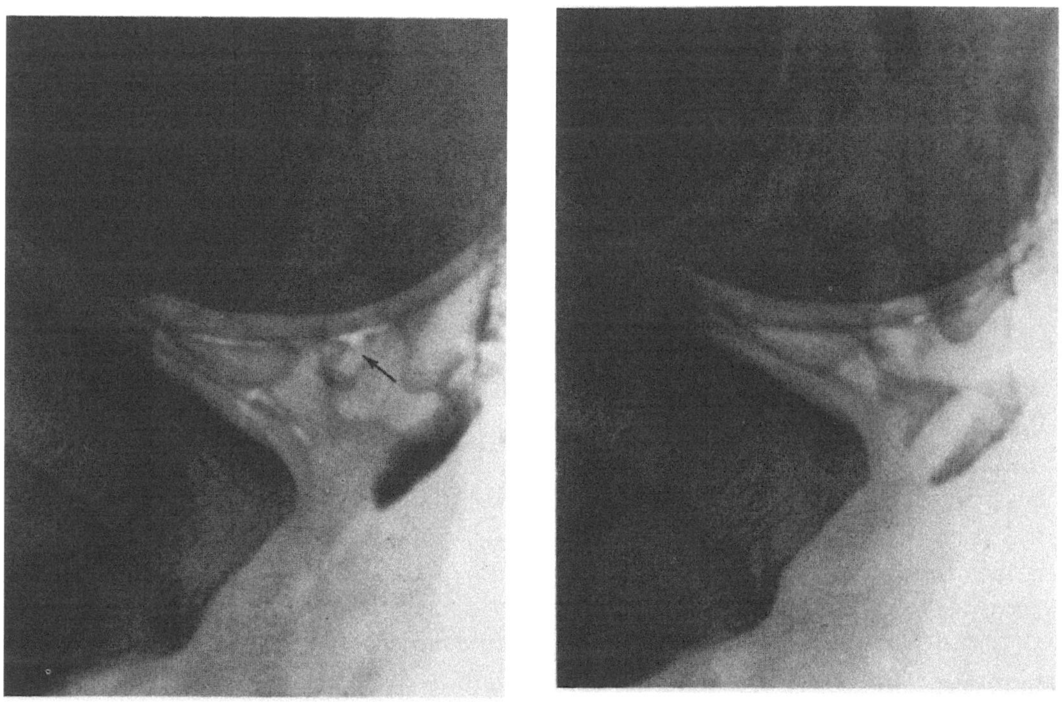

Fig. 161. Longitudinal rupture of posterior medial horn. Semimembranous bursa. Communication between bursa and articular cavity superposed on meniscal periphery (*arrow*)

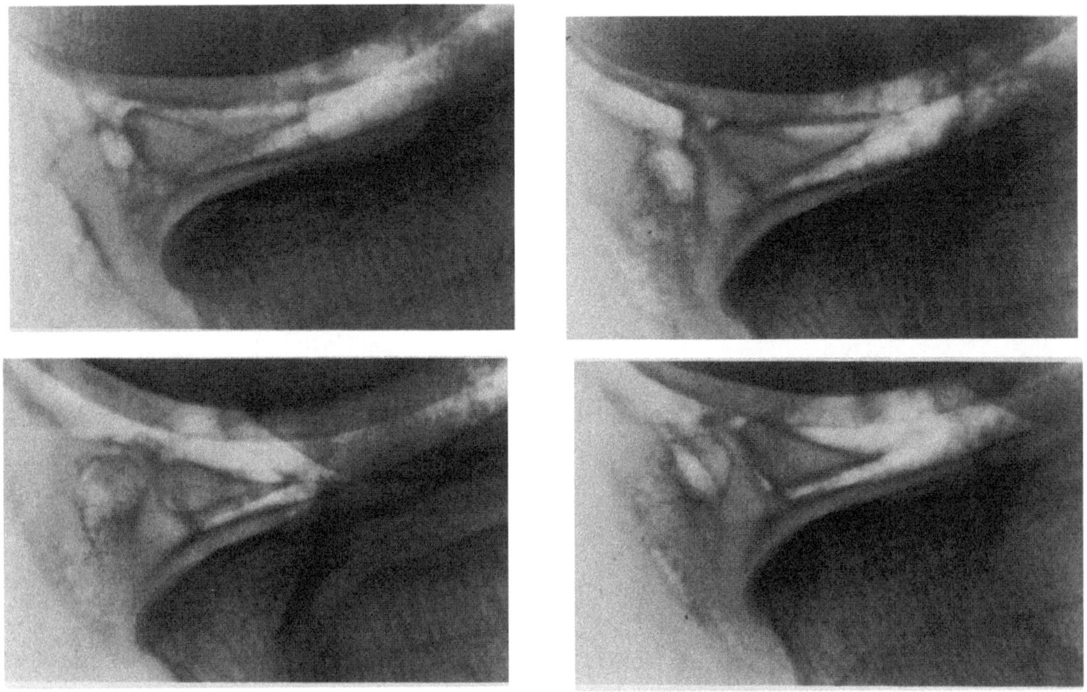

Fig. 162. Longitudinal rupture of posterior medial horn. Semimembranous bursa. Communication between bursa and articular cavity superposed on meniscal periphery

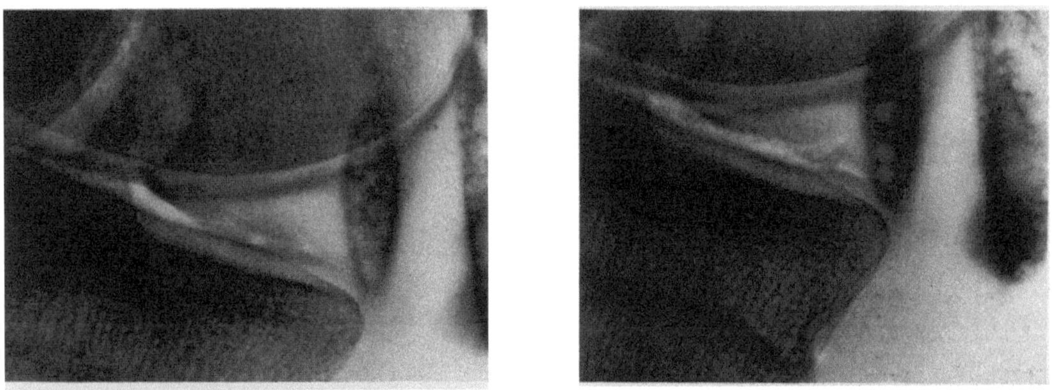

Fig. 163. Tangential incisure of posterior medial horn on the inferior side. Semimembranosogastrocnemial bursa

ness of the bursae, differentiation is not very important. The transition from the semimembranous bursa to the articular cavity is localized at a lower level, and the aperture of the bursa can be projected at the level of the medial posterior horn (Figs. 161, 162, and 164). Since Adams published the first article on these bursae in 1840, extensive literature on this subject has accumulated. Dilatation of the semimembranosogastrocnemial bursa has been described under various synonyms, e.g., popliteal cyst, synovial cyst, and Baker cyst. Baker defined the cysts he described

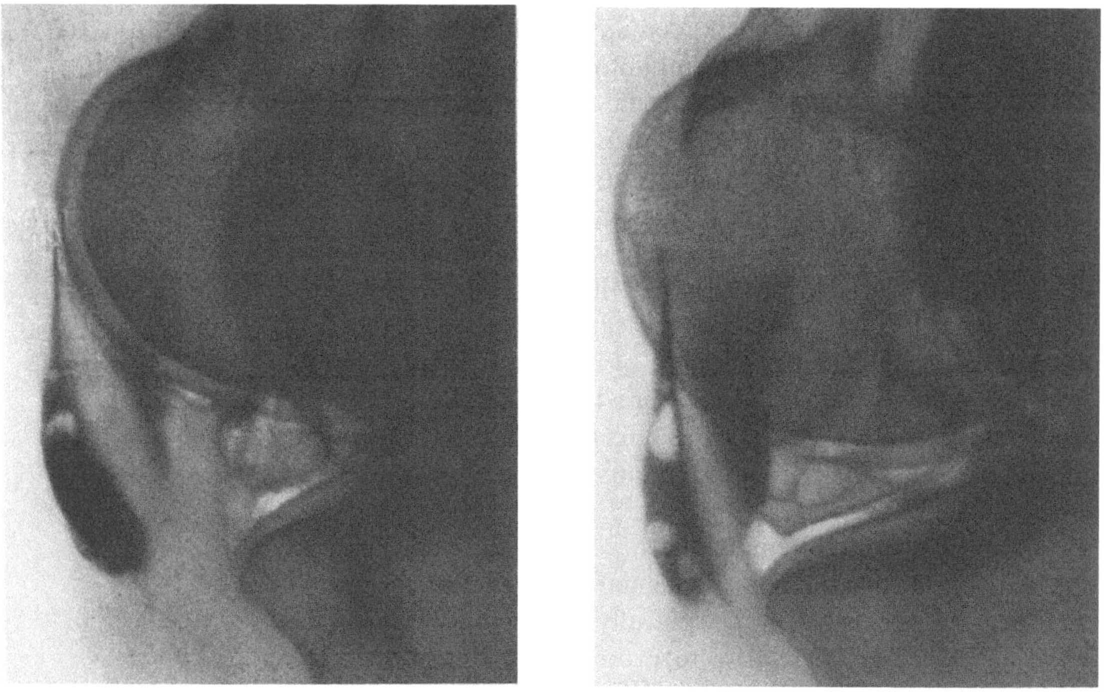

Fig. 164. Mainly filling of the semimembranosogastrocnemial bursa. The communication between semimembranous bursa and articular cavity is also clearly visible

as a herniation of the synovial membrane through a defect of the joint capsule. Wilson's study (1938) would seem to warrant the conclusion that 50% of normal individuals have a semimembranosogastrocnemial bursa which communicates with the articular cavity. Olsen (1967) and Freiberger et al. (1966) found filling of the bursa in 20% of their arthrograms. These authors concluded that abnormal enlargement of the bursa constitutes a "Baker cyst."

Several authors have attempted to indicate the difference between the asymptomatic semimembranosogastrocnemial bursa found by arthrography and the clinical cyst found in the popliteal fossa in some patients. Doppman (1965) concluded that the presence of an enlarged semimembranosogastrocnemial bursa is not the same thing as the presence of a clinically evident cyst. In actual practice this means that the finding of a bursa filled with contrast medium does not mean that the patient should have symptoms which cause any discomfort. Nor is it always possible to find such a bursa by clinical examination. If clinical examination discloses an unmistakable Baker cyst, and arthrography reveals an enlarged semimembranosogastrocnemial bursa, the correlation can be accepted as unmistakable.

As Wolfe and Ben Colloff (1972) demonstrated, two patients can have an equally large semimembranosogastrocnemial bursa; while one patient is asymptomatic, the other shows the typical features of a Baker cyst. Studies by Pavlov et al. (1977) of cadaver knees revealed that the communication between articular cavity and semimembranosogastrocnemial bursa can vary widely in size. It seems likely that, given an ample communication between articular cavity and bursa, the latter fills with contrast medium at arthrography. When the communication is narrow this may not be the case, unless the presence of a large amount of intra-articular fluid so dilates the aperture that filling of the bursa is observed. Not infrequently the bursa is filled only with air; this could indicate a narrow communication between articular cavity and bursa.

To summarize, in many individuals, a normal communication between semimembranosogastrocnemial bursa and articular cavity is present, although arthrographically not demonstrable unless intra-articular lesions give rise to protracted hydrops. Such lesions are meniscal lesions, degenerative lesions of the articular cartilage, corpora libera, cruciate ligament ruptures, patellar chondropathy, and inflammations such as rheumatoid arthritis (Figs. 153 and 161–163). The radiologist should mention in his report that the presence of a semimembranosogastrocnemial bursa of specified size has been established. The designation Baker cyst can be confusing and should preferably be avoided. Baker cyst is primarily a clinical diagnosis.

In the majority of patients, a lesion of one of the intra-articular structures should be demonstrable in addition to the clinical diagnosis. Our own investigation into associated intra-articular lesions confirmed this. Of 122 patients with a semimembranosogastrocnemial bursa which has an inferior margin extending past the tibial plateau, only 29 had no demonstrable intra-articular lesions (Table 11).

Table 11. Intra-articular pathology in the presence of a large semimembranosogastrocnemial bursa (with an inferior delimitation extending distal to the tibial plateau)

No abnormalities found	29
Meniscal lesions	49
Chondropathia patellae	28
After meniscectomy	11
Ruptured cruciate ligaments	4
Rheumatoid arthritis	1
Number of patients	122

Table 11 shows that meniscal lesions and patellar chondropathy were frequently found in association with a large semimembranosogastrocnemial bursa. The bursa can be particularly enlarged in rheumatoid arthritis, when its lower margin can extend as far as the calf (Fig. 153). Rupture of a markedly enlarged bursa can give to a pattern of symptoms reminiscent of deep-seated thrombosis in the calf. In such patients (usually suffering from rheumatoid arthritis), arthrography can confirm the diagnosis. The conclusion that, in view of the size of the bursa, a Baker cyst should be clinically demonstrable in the patient is erroneous.

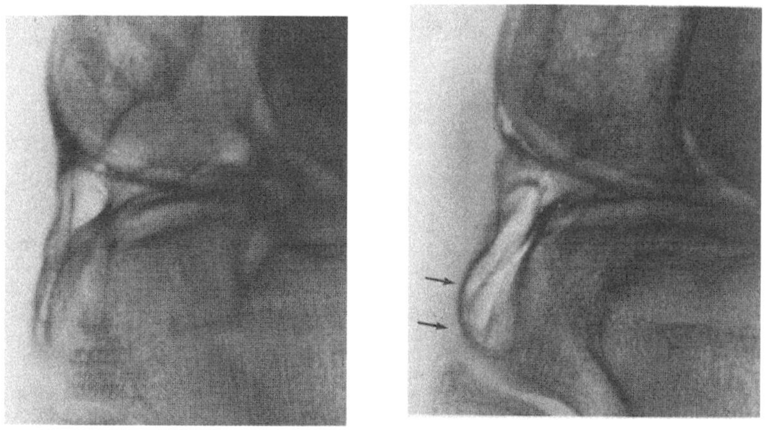

a

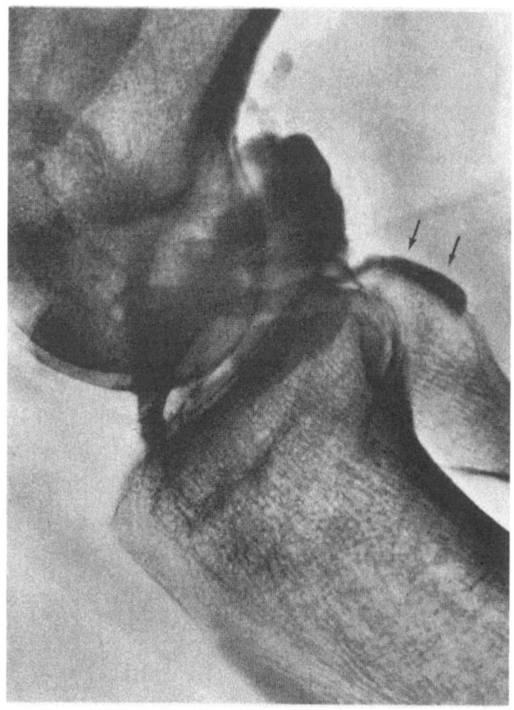

b

Fig. 165a and b. Popliteal bursa (a) extending to just above the tibiofibular joint (*arrows*). Popliteal bursa (b) extending to behind the tibiofibular joint (*arrows*)

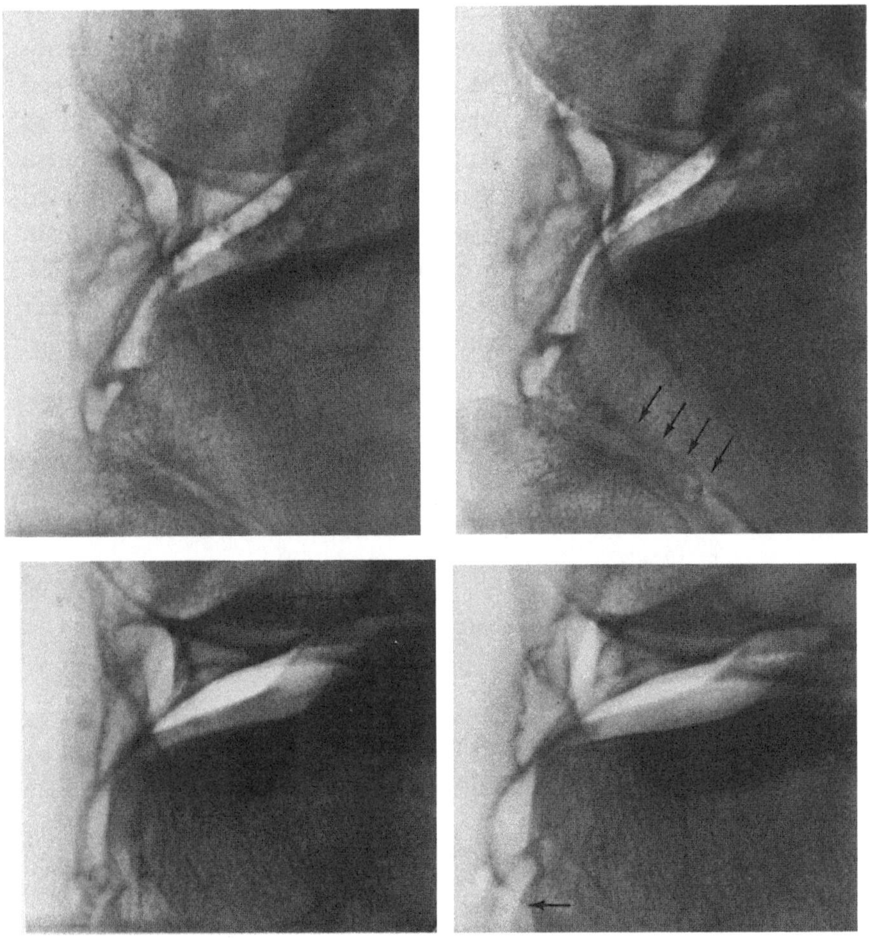

a

b

Fig. 166a and b. Two patients (a, b). Stereoscopic photographs. Communication between popliteal bursa and tibiofibular joint (*arrows*)

6.2.3 Popliteal Bursa

This bursa, localized between the posterior aspect of the tibia and the popliteus muscle, can extend behind the tibiofibular joint, with which it regularly communicates (Figs. 165 and 166). On the superior side, the bursa communicates with the articular cavity via an ample tubular structure around the popliteal tendon.

7 Lesions of the Articular Cartilage

7.1 General Aspects

Studies by Collins (1949) and MacCall (1969) have shown that the articular cartilage can be divided into four layers. The superficial layer consists of collagenous fibers arranged parallel to the articular surface and lies on top of a cartilage layer of disc-shaped cartilage cells. The collagenous fibers in this layer form an irregular network. In the third layer the collagenous fibers are arranged more perpendicular to the articular surface, while the cartilage cells are of circular shape and arranged in clusters. The fourth layer contains some calcium and is adjacent to the subchondral bone.

In Sect. 4.2 has discussed the nutrition and the properties of the cartilage as well as the histologic changes found in the case of degeneration were discussed. This description applies not only to patellar chondropathy, but also to cartilage degeneration elsewhere in the knee joint. Chondropathy should be regarded as incipient arthrosis deformans and is not a separate entity. In the case of arthrotic lesions of the knee joint, the cartilage shows varying degrees of destruction. In the event of total local destruction of the articular cartilage, osteosclerosis develops at the site affected, and at the periphery of the joint osteophytes of cancellous bone develop. Moreover, cysts may be present in the area affected.

7.2 Etiology and Double Contrast Arthrography

In the majority of cases, arthrotic lesions of the knee joint can be explained on the basis of an existing intra-articular pathology. In the following sections, a primary and a secondary form of arthrosis deformans are discussed.

7.2.1 Primary Form

Various congenital anomalies characterized by a deficient or poor primordial development of articular cartilage can lead to premature arthrosis deformans. Anomalies of possible importance in this respect include multiple epiphyseal dysplasia, spondyloepiphyseal dysplasia, Morquio-Brailsford disease, and other anomalies. On the other hand, isolated dysplasias of the tibiofemoral and the patellofemoral joint can give rise to abnormal pressures, thus causing arthrotic lesions. Such dysplasias have already been mentioned in the discussion of patellar chondropathy.

7.2.2 Secondary Form

In the secondary form, the arthrotic lesions result from a recent or longstanding intra-articular pathology.

7.2.2.1 Direct Injury

During a traumatic impact on the knee joint, not only can lesions of the femur, patella, or tibia occur, but in many cases the

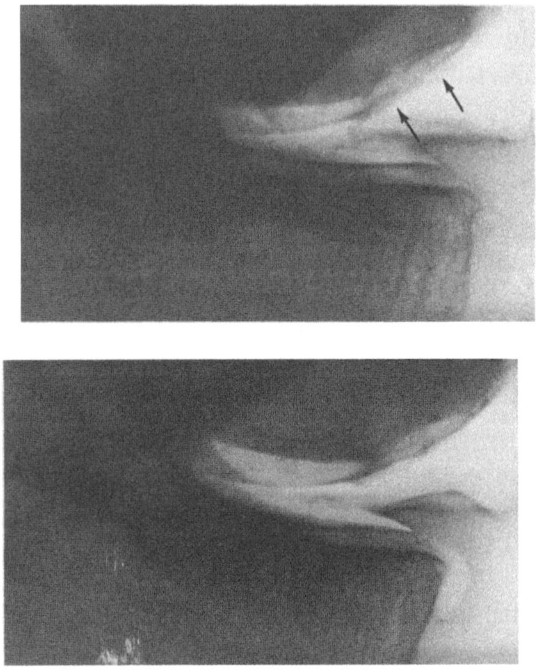

Fig. 167. Condition after old fracture of femoral condyle. Arthrography: degeneration of cartilage of the femoral condyle (*arrows*)

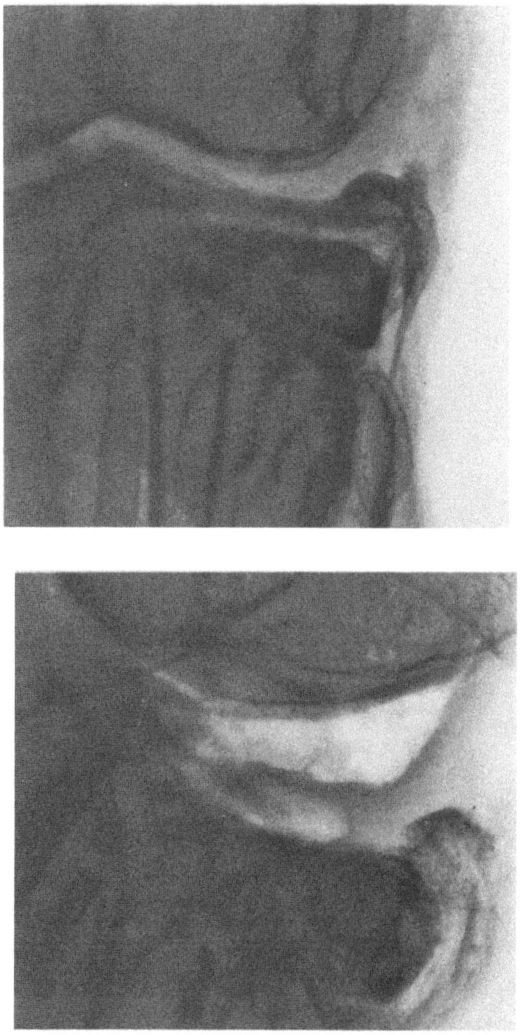

Fig. 168. Condition after operation for giant-cell tumor of the proximal part of the tibia. Marked degenerative lesions in the lateral intra-articular space. Articular cartilage narrowed. Marked degenerative lesions of the lateral meniscus

articular cartilage is also injured. Such damage can be demonstrated by double contrast arthrography (Fig. 167; also Figs. 96 and 97). After an operation in the immediate vicinity of the articular cavity, the normal situation can obviously be so influenced that the osseous and cartilaginous boundaries are severely disturbed, so that arthrotic lesions result (Fig. 168).

7.2.2.2 Indirect Injury

Meniscal Lesions. Recurrent incarcerations in the case of longstanding meniscal lesions can cause damage in particular to the

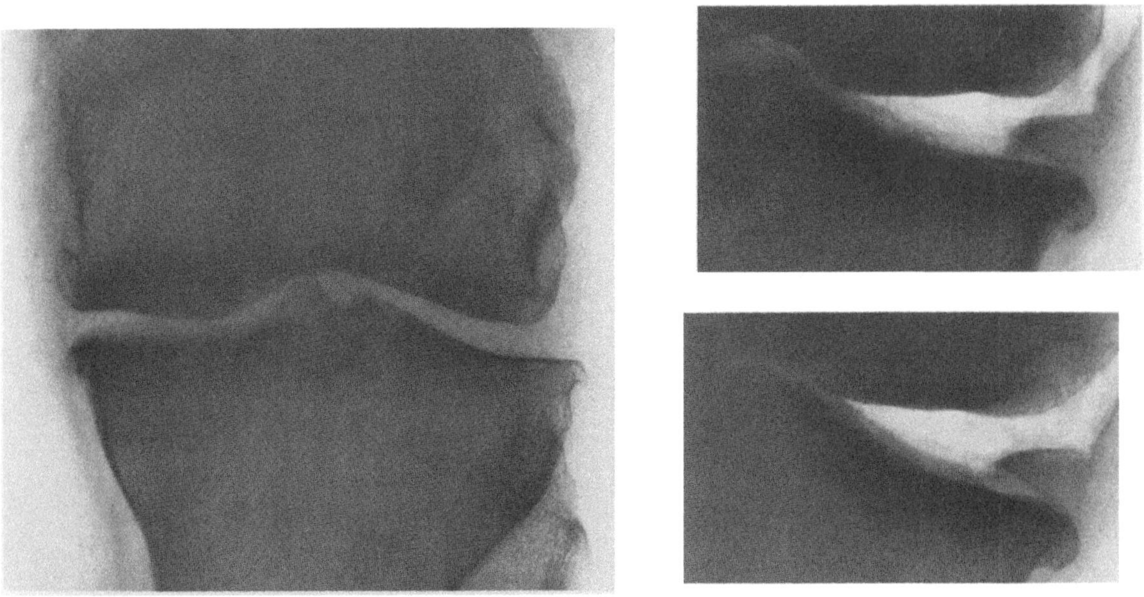

Fig. 169. Condition 20 years after traumatic injury. Severe arthrosis deformans. Cartilage of the femoral condyle destroyed. Degenerative lesions of the medial meniscus

cartilage of the femoral condyle (Fig. 169; also Figs. 67 and 70). The necessity of radiologic examination following meniscectomy has already been pointed out in the chapter on meniscal lesions (Sect. 3.6.4). After total excision of the meniscus the regenerate is usually of regular shape.

A regenerate does not protect from degeneration of the articular cartilage. According to King (1936), postoperative cartilage degeneration is proportional in severity to the extent of the meniscectomy. Partial meniscectomy, therefore, would be preferable to total meniscectomy.

Clinical and radiologic signs of arthrosis deformans of the knee after meniscectomy are reported in the literature to be found in about 25% of cases (Uebermuth, 1941; Lagergren, 1945). Since the introduction of arthroscopy, less marked degenerative cartilage lesions can also be demonstrated. For example Jackson (1968) found cartilage degeneration after meniscectomy in 21%–67% of cases. The largest percentages were found after the longest postoperative observation periods. Since the duration of the preoperative history did not prove to influence the incidence of the lesions, Jackson considered it improbable that a ruptured meniscus in situ could be the primary cause of the radiologic changes observed. In his opinion the causative factor was to be found precisely in the loss of the meniscus. On the basis of this conclusion he urged that a conservative operative technique be used.

Fig. 170. Situation after meniscectomy. Arthrography: probably regenerate. No more than slight degeneration of this structure. Marked degenerative lesions of femoral cartilage, and local deep defect (*arrow*). See page 143, Fig. 171

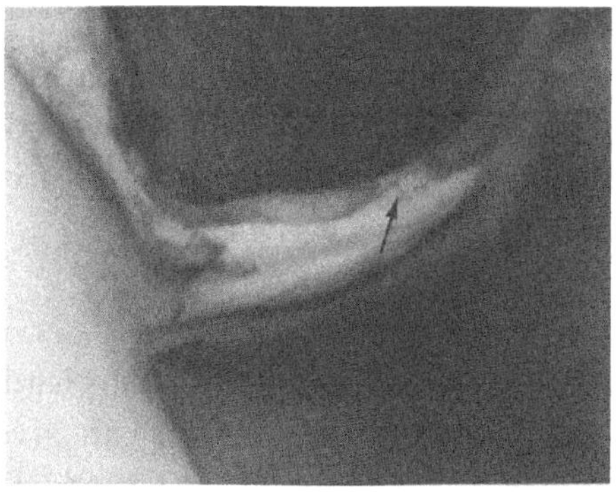

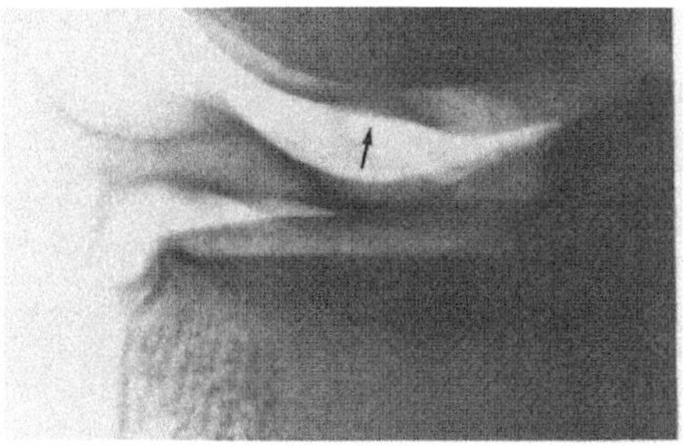

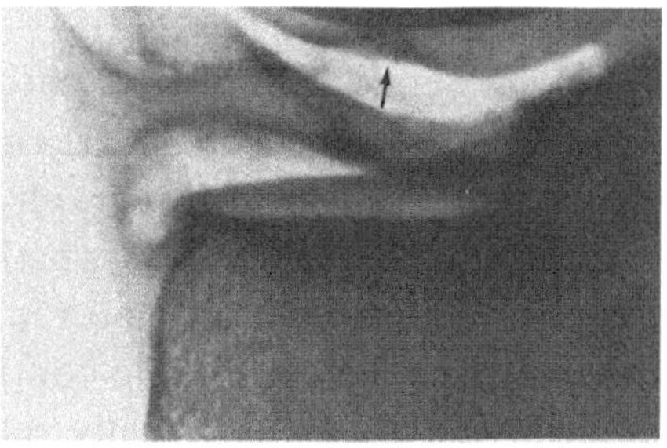

Fig. 172. Stereoscopic photographs of the lateral intra-articular space after old rupture of the collateral ligament. Intra-articular space dilatated; meniscus intact; local defect of cartilage of femoral condyle (*arrows*)

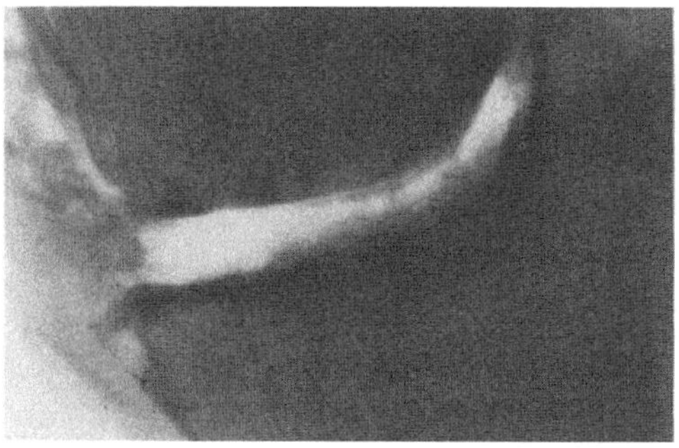

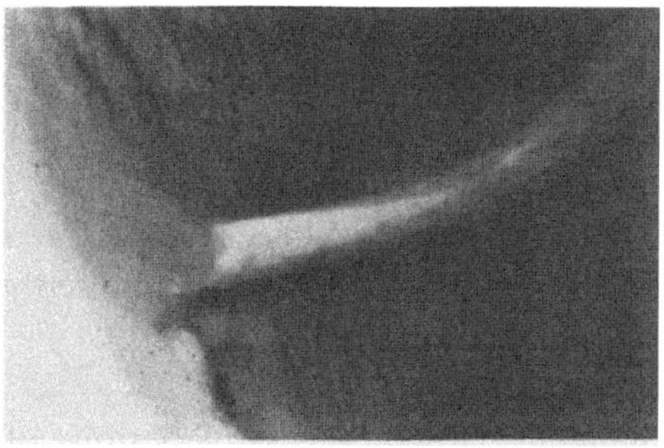

Fig. 173. Rheumatoid arthritis. Distinct synovitis. Almost complete destruction of articular cartilage

Whenever ruptured meniscal remnants remain in situ, extensive degenerative lesions of the articular cartilage can develop in the long run. The arthrographically visualized cartilage defects can be very clearly demonstrated by arthroscopy (Figs. 170 and 171 see page 143; also Fig. 74).

Cruciate and Collateral Ligament Lesions. Long-standing lesions of the ligamentous apparatus can lead to marked instability of the knee joint, which in turn can give rise to degeneration of the articular cartilage (Fig. 172).

Osteochondritis Dissecans. This form of aseptic osteonecrosis of the knee joint is characterized by an irregular contour of the articular cartilage at the site of the osteochondritic focus. The cartilage at this site is indented, and degenerative lesions can be present.

Inflammations. Septic arthritis, like chronic rheumatoid arthritis, leads to severe destruction of the articular cartilage. These types of arthritis rarely call for arthrography, but in the presence of rheumatoid arthritis, the question whether a ruptured Baker cyst is present can be an indication for arthrography. In patients with rheumatoid arthritis, double contrast arthrography reveals marked synovitis as well as usually reduced and locally absent articular cartilage. Apart from the reduced articular cavity and the degeneration of cartilage, there are arthrotic lesions such as peripheral sclerosis, small cysts, and hook formation (Fig. 173; also Fig. 111).

Changed Pressures. Consolidation of a low femoral fracture in a nonoptimal position can so alter the pressures within the knee joint that some parts of the articular cartilage are subject to excessive stress. This gives rise to degenerative lesions (Van Duyn, 1977). In a similar way degenerative lesions in the patellofemoral joint result from dislocations of the quadriceps tendon (Figs. 96 and 97). Whether obesity per se sufficiently increases the pressure on the articular cartilage to give rise to degenerative lesions is not readily demonstrable. However, in combination with other causative factors, obesity can undoubtedly contribute to the etiology of such lesions.

Hemophilia. How degenerative lesions of the articular cartilage develop in hemophilia is not exactly known. The pathologically changed synovial membrane growing over the cartilage can unfavorably influence the nutrition of the cartilage, and destruction might result. It has been experimentally demonstrated that degenerative lesions of the cartilage cannot be produced by repeated intra-articular injections of blood. In hemophilia there is no indication for double contrast arthrography. The arthrotic lesions are clearly visible in the skeleton. The articular cavity of the patellofemoral joint is usually markedly reduced because the patellar cartilage is almost completely overgrown and disappears (Fig. 112). In subsequent stages of the disease there may be ankylosis of the patellofemoral joint and even of the tibiofemoral joint (Forrai, 1976; Driessen, 1973).

Metabolic Disorders. Articular chondrocalcinosis can be a symptom of ochronosis and hyperparathyroidism. Primary articular chondrocalcinosis also occurs as pseudogout. These diseases can cause arthrosis deformans. Uratic arthritis is another metabolic disorder which can cause degenerative lesions of the knee joint. Arthrography is rarely indicated in any of these conditions, except as an aid in the diagnosis of traumatic articular lesions.

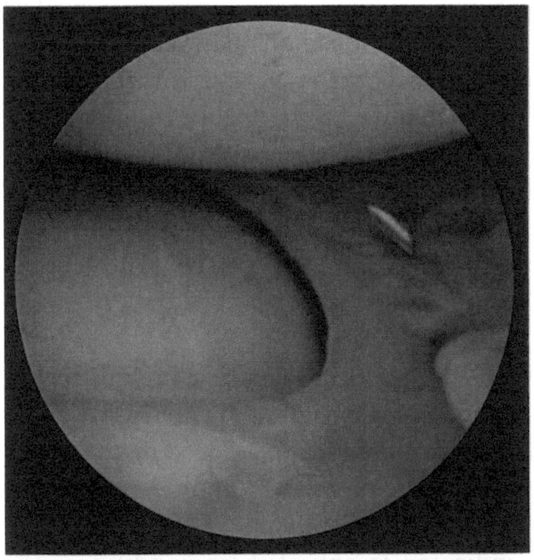

Fig. 77. Arthroscopy (Eikelaar). Normal medial meniscus. The visible needle can be used to establish whether part of the meniscus can be luxated

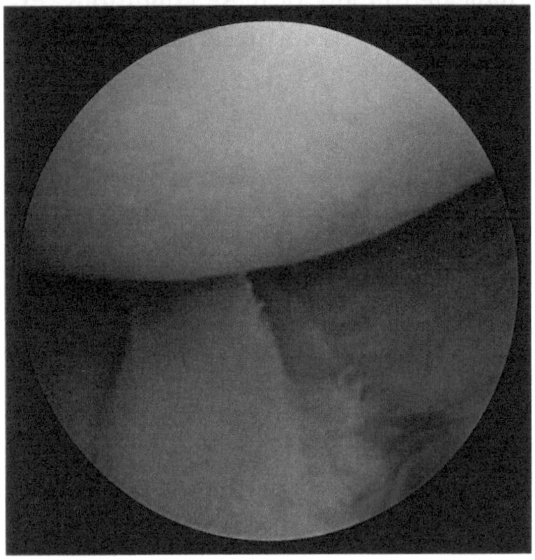

Fig. 78. Longitudinal rupture of the medial meniscus (arthroscopic photograph: Eikelaar)

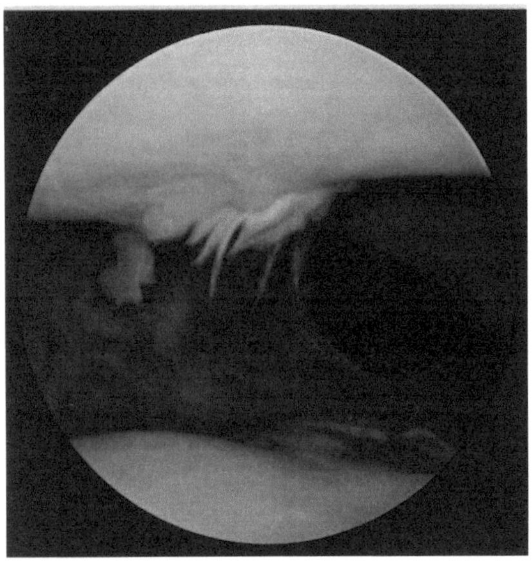

Fig. 87. Arthroscopy (Eikelaar). Patellar chondropathy. Shreds of degenerated cartilage are visible near the linea eminens

Fig. 124. Arthroscopy. Visualization of the anterior cruciate ligament. Synovial membrane, adipose tissue and femoral condyle are clearly visible

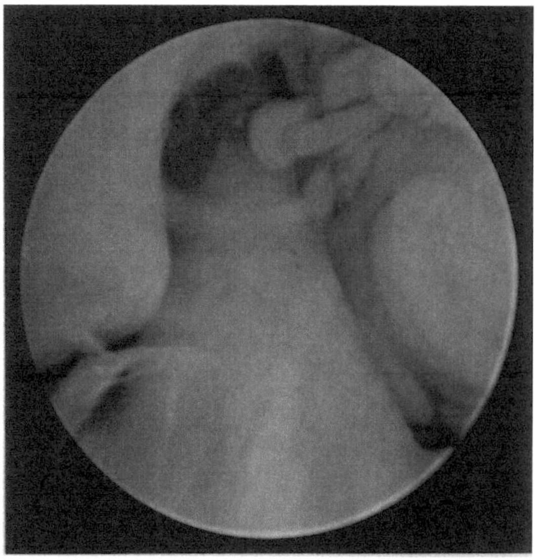

Fig. 150c. Arthroscopy: Hoffa flake clearly visible. Agreement with arthrographic findings

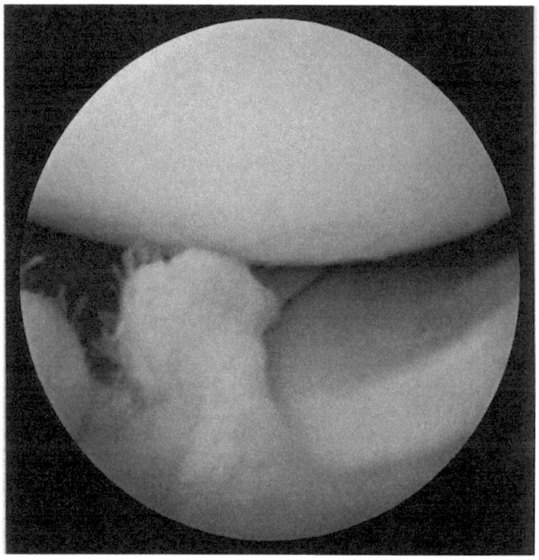

Fig. 171. The same patient as in Fig. 170. Arthroscopy: marked degenerative lesions of the femoral condyle. Area of complete destruction of cartilage clearly visible (Eikelaar)

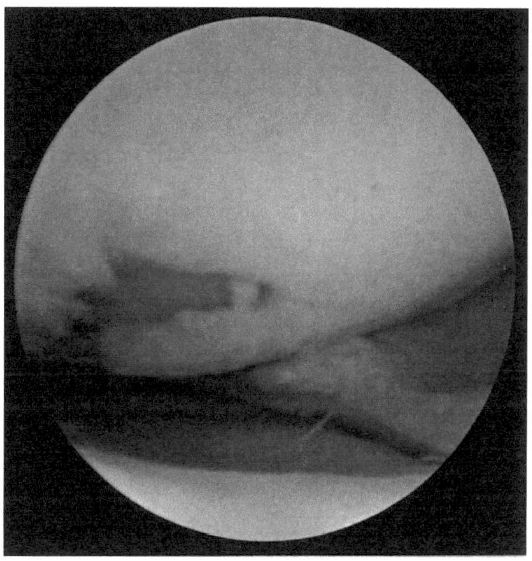

References

Adams, R., Dublin, J.: Chronic rheumatoid arthritis of the knee joint. Med. Science **17**, 520 (1840)

Andren, L., Wehlin, L.: Double-contrast arthrography of the knee with horizontal Roentgen ray beam. Acta Orthop. Scand. **29**, 307–314 (1960)

Angell, F.L.: Fluoroscopic technique of double contrast arthrography of the knee. Radiol. Clin. North Am. **9/1** pag. 85–98 (1971)

Archer, C.R., Yeager, V.: Internal structures of the knee visualized by computed tomography. J. Comp. Ax. Tom. **2**, 181–183 (1978)

Baker, W.M.: Formation of synovial cysts in the leg in connection with disease in the knee joint. St. Bartholomew's Hosp. Rep. **13**, 245 (1877)

Bandi, W.: Chondromalacia patellae und femoropatellare Arthrose. Helv. Chir. Acta [Suppl.] **2**, 1–70 (1972)

Bandi, W.: Zur Frage der traumatischen Auslösung der Chondromalacia patellae. Orthopäde **3**, 201–207 (1974)

Bandi, W., Brennwald, J.: The significance of femoropatellar pressure in the pathogenesis and treatment of chondromalacia patellae and femoropatellar arthrosis. The Knee Joint. Proceedings of the International Congress, Sept. 1973

Baumgartl, F.: Das Kniegelenk. Berlin-Heidelberg-New York: Springer 1964

Benninghoff, A.: Form und Bau der Gelenkknorpel in ihren Beziehungen zur Function. Z. Zellforsch. Mikr. Anat. **2**, 782–862 (1925)

Bessler, W.: Die Röntgensymptome der Synovitis villosa des Kniegelenks. Fortschr. Röntgenstr. **99**, 343–353 (1963)

Bircher, E.: Pneumoradiographie des Knies und der anderen Gelenke. Schweiz. Med. Wochenschr. **61**, 1210–1211 (1931)

Bircher, E.: Über Binnenverletzungen des Kniegelenks. Arch. Clin. Chir. **177**, 290–359 (1933)

Bircher, E., Oberholzer, J.: Die Kniegelenkkapsel im Pneumoradiographiebilde. Acta Radiol. **15**, 452–466 (1934)

Blumensaat, C.: Die Lageabweichungen und Verrenkungen der Kniescheibe. Ergebnisse der Chirurgie und Orthopädie **31**, 149–223 (1938)

Bollet, A.J., Nance, J.L.: Chondroitin sulfate concentration and chain length, water and ash content. J. Clin. Invest. **45**, 1170–1177 (1966)

Bonnin, J.G.: Cysts of the semilunar cartilages of the knee joint. Br. J. Surg. **40**, 558–565 (1953)

Boyd, D.: Knee joint visualization. Roentgenographic study with iopax. J. Bone Joint Surg. **16**, 671–680 (1934)

Brantigan, O.C., Voshell, F.: The mechanics of the ligaments and menisci of the knee joint. J. Bone Joint Surg. **23**, 44–65 (1941)

Brantigan, O.C., Voshell, F.: The tibial collateral ligament: its function, its bursae, and its relation to the medial meniscus. J. Bone Joint Surg. **25**, 123–131 (1943)
Brattström, H.: Shape of the intercondylar groove normally and in recurrent dislocation of patella. Acta Orthop. Scand. [Suppl.] **68**, pag. 1–148 (1964)
Büdinger, K.: Über Ablösung von Gelenkteilen und verwandte Prozesse. Dtsch. Z. Chir. **84**, 311–365 (1906)
Büdinger, K.: Über traumatische Knorpelrisse im Kniegelenk. Dtsch. Z. Chir. **92**, 510–536 (1908)
Butt, W.P., McIntyre, J.L.: Double contrast Arthrography of the Knee. Radiology **92**, 487–499 (1969)
Bywaters, E.G.L.: The metabolism of joint tissues. J. Pathol. Bacteriol. **44**, 247–268 (1937)
Collins, D.H.: The Pathology of Articular and Spinal Diseases, p. 74–115. London: Arnold 1949
Collins, D.H., McElligott, T.F.: Sulphate ($^{35}SO_4$) uptake by chondrocytes in relation to histological changes in osteoarthritic human articular cartilage. Ann. Rheum. Dis. **19**, 318–330 (1960)
Dalinka, M.K., Garofola, J.: The infrapatellar synovial fold: A cause for confusion in the evaluation of the anterior cruciate ligament. Am. J. Roentgenol. **127**, 589–591 (1976)
Debnam, J.W., Staple, T.W.: Arthrography of the knee after meniscectomy. Radiology **113**, 67–71 (1974)
Doppman, J.L.: Baker's cyst and the normal gastrocnemio-semimembranosus bursa. Am. J. Roentgenol. **94**, 646–652 (1965)
Driessen, A.P.P.M.: Arthropaties in Haemophiliacs. Groningen: Thesis 1973
Duyn, C.D. van: Fracturen van het distale deel van het femur. Groningen: Thesis 1977
Eikelaar, H.R.: Arthroscopy of the knee. Groningen: Thesis 1975
Ekholm, R.: Nutrition of articular cartilage. Acta Anat. **24**, 329–338 (1955)
Fagerberg, S.: Tomographic studies of the normal and injured knee. Acta Radiol. [Suppl.] **138**, 1–93 (1956)
Fairbank, T.J.: Knee joint changes after meniscectomy. J. Bone Joint Surg. **30B/4**, 664–670 (1948)
Ficat, P.: L'arthrographie opaque de genou. p. 243. Paris: Masson 1957
Ficat, P.: Pathologie des menisques et des ligaments du genou. p. 285. Paris: Masson 1962
Ficat, P.: Pathologie femoro-patellaire. Paris: Masson 1970a
Ficat, P.: Les Déséquilibres Rotuliens. Paris: Masson 1973
Ficat, P., Philippe, J., Bizou, H.: Le défilé fémoro-patellaire. Rev. Med. Toulouse **6**, 241–244 (1970b)
Fischedick, O.: Die Kontrastdarstellung des Kniegelenkes nach Meniscektomie. Fortschr. Röntgenstr. **99**, 685–692 (1963)
Fischedick, O.: Veränderungen des hinteren Anteils der Kniegelenkskapsel im Arthrogramm. Chirurg **40**, 408–411 (1969a)
Fischedick, O.: Welchen Wert hat die Kniegelenksarthrographie? Z. Orthop. **106**, 759–765 (1969b)
Fischedick, O.: Zur Pathologie des Band- und Kapselapparates des Kniegelenkes im Arthrogramm. Fortschr. Röntgenstr. **115**, 312–320 (1971)

Fischedick, O., Socha, P.: Indikation und Ergebnisse der Kontrastdarstellung des Kniegelenkes mit positivem Kontrastmittel. Chirurg **31**, 13–19 (1960a)
Fischedick, O., Socha, P.: Erfahrungen bei der Arthrographie des Kniegelenkes mit positivem Kontrastmittel. Röntgenblätter **13**, 337–344 (1960b)
Fischer, L.P., Guyot, J., Gonon, G.P., Coucelles, P., Dahhan, P.: Du rôle des muscles et des ligaments dans le contrôle de la stabilité du genou. Anatomia Clinica **1**, 1–11 (1978)
Forrai, J.: Radiology of Haemophilic Arthropathies. Budapest: Akadémiai Kiadó 1976
Freeman, M.A.R.: The pathogenesis of primary osteoarthrosis: an hypothesis. In: Modern Trends in Orthopedic. Graham Apley, A. (ed.), pp. 40–94. London: Butterworths 1972
Freeman, M.A.R.: Adult Articular Cartilage. London: Isaac Pitman 1973
Freiberger, R.H., Killoran, P.J., Cardona, G.: Arthrography of the knee by double contrast method. Am. J. Roentgenol. **97**, 736–747 (1966)
Fürmaier, A.: Beitrag zur Mechanik der Patella und des Gesamt-Kniegelenkes. Arch. Orthop. Unfallchir. **46**, 78–90 (1953a)
Fürmaier, A.: Beitrag zur Ätiologie der Chondropathia patellae. Arch. Orthop. Unfallchir. **46**, 178–196 (1953b)
Gaillard, J.M.: Les Menisques de l'articulation du genou. Etude morphologique et fonctionelle. Arch. Anat. (Strasbourg) **49**, 327–357 (1966)
Green, W.T.: Painfull Bipartite patellae. Clin. Orthop. **110**, 197–200 (1975)
Griffiths, H.J., D'Orsi, C.J.: Use of Xerography in cruciate Ligament Injuries. Am. J. Roentgenol. **121**, 94–96 (1974)
Gschwend, N., Bischofsberger, R.J.: Die Chondropathia patellae. Praxis **60**, 562–572 (1971)
Hall, F.M.: Pitfalls in knee arthrography. Radiology **118**,55–62 (1976)
Harkness, R.D.: Mechanical Properties of Collagenous Tissues. In: Treatise on Collagen, Part A. Gould, B.S. (ed.). London-New York: Academic Press 1968
Heinold, G. von: Erfahrungen und Operationsergebnisse von 455 Meniskusschäden bei Bergleuten. Beitr. Orthop. Traumatol. **12**, 418–423 (1965)
Henssge, J.: Die Arthrosis deformans des Patellagleitweges. Zentralbl. Chir. **87**, 1381–1387 (1962)
Hodge, J., McKibbin, B.: The Nutrition of mature and immature joint cartilage in rabbits. J. Bone Joint Surg. **51B**, 140–147 (1969)
Honner, R., Thompson, R.C.: The nutritional pathways or articular cartilage. J. Bone Joint Surg. **53A**, 742–748 (1971)
Hugston, J.C.: Subluxation of the patella. J. Bone Joint Surg. **50A**, 1003–1026 (1968)
Insall, J., Salvati, E.: Patella position in the normal knee joint. Radiology **101**, 101–104 (1971)
Jackson, J.P.: Contribution to a discussion. J. Bone Joint Surg. **49B**, 584 (1967)
Jackson, J.P.: Degenerative changes in the knee after meniscectomy. Br. Med. J. **2**, 525–527 (1968)

Jackson, R.W., Abe, I.: The role of arthroscopy in the management of disorders of the knee. J. Bone Joint Surg. **54B**, 310–322 (1972)
Jackson, R.W., De Haven, K.E.: Arthroscopy of the knee. Clin. Orthop. **107**, 87–92 (1975)
Jelaso, D.V., Usar, Mc.: Positive contrast arthrography of the knee. Am. J. Roentgenol. **103**, 669–673 (1968)
Jonasch, E.: Auftreten von Knochenveränderungen bei Zysten des lateralen Meniskus des Kniegelenkes. Fortschr. Röntgenstr. **93**, 466–471 (1960)
Kaplan, E.B.: The embryology of the menisci of the knee joint. Bull. Hosp. Joint Dis. (N.Y.) **16**, 111–124 (1955)
Kaplan, E.B.: Discoid lateral meniscus of the knee joint. Nature, mechanism, and operative treatment. J. Bone Joint Surg. **39A**, 77–87 (1957)
Kaplan, E.B.: Some aspects of functional anatomy of the human knee-joint. Clin. Orthop. **23**, 18–29 (1962)
Katzberg, R.W., Burgener, F.A., Fischer, H.W.: Evaluation of various contrast agents for improved arthography. Invest. Radiology **11**, 528–533 (1976)
King, D.: The function of semilunar cartilages. J. Bone Joint Surg. **18/4**, 1069–1076 (1936)
Kingma, M.J.: De letsels van de menisci van het kniegewricht. Ned. T. Geneesk. **99/2**, 1229–1246 (1955)
Kiss, J., Moir, J.D.: Experience with arthrographic examination of the knee joint. J. Can. Assoc. Radiol. **19**, 187–191 (1968)
Kleinberg, S.: Pulmonary embolism following oxygen injection of the knee. J.A.M.A. **89**, 172–173 (1927)
Lagergren, K.A.: Meniscus operations and secondary arthrosis deformans. Acta Orthopaedica **14/4**, 280–289 (1945)
Lanz, T. v., Wachsmuth, W.: Praktische Anatomie, Bd. I, Teil 4. Berlin-Heidelberg-New York: Springer 1972
Last, R.J.: Some anatomical details of the knee joint. J. Bone Joint Surg. **30B**, 683–688 (1948)
Last, R.J.: The popliteus muscle and the lateral meniscus. J. Bone Joint Surg. **32B/1**, 93–99 (1950)
Leroux, G., Collette, J.M.: Arthrographie opaque et mixte simultanée du genou. Etude compérative des images. J. Radiol. Electrol. **41**, 355–358 (1960)
Liljedahl, S.O., Lindvall, N., Wetterfors, J.: Roentgendiagnosis of rupture of anterior cruciate ligament. Acta Radiol. [Diagn.] (Stockh.) **4**, 225–239 (1966)
Lindblom, K.: The arthrographic appearance of the ligaments of the knee. Acta Radiol. (Stockh.) **19**, 582–600 (1938)
Lindblom, K.: Arthrography of the knee. Roentgenographic and anatomic study. Acta Radiol [Suppl.] (Stockh.) **74**, 1–112 (1948)
Linn, F.C.: Lubrication of Animal Joints. 2. The Mechanism. J. Biol. **1**, 193–198 (1968)
Linn, F.C., Sokoloff, L.: Movement and composition of interstitial fluid of cartilage. Arthritis Rheum. **8**, 481–494 (1965)
Maquet, P.G.J.: Biomechanics of the Knee. Berlin-Heidelberg-New York: Springer 1976
Maldague, B., Malghem, J.: Le faux profil rotulien ou profil vrai des facettes rotuliennes. Ann. Radiol. (Paris) **19** (6), 573–581 (1976)

Maroudas, A.: Physiochemical Properties of Cartilage in the Light of Ion-exchange theory. Biophys. J. **8**, 575–595 (1968a)

Maroudas, A., Bullough, P., Swanson, S.A.V., Freeman, M.A.R.: The permeability of articular cartilage. J. Bone Joint Surg. **50B**, 166–177 (1968b)

McBeath, A.A., Wirka, H.W.: Positive contrast arthrography of the knee. Clin. Orthop. **88**, 70–75 (1972)

McCall, J.G.: Load deformation response of the microstructure of articular cartilage. In: Lubrication and Wear in Joints. Wright, V. (ed.), p. 152–205. Leeds: Sector Publishing 1969

McConaill, M.A.: The function of intra-articular fibrocartilages with special references to the knee and inferior radio-ulnar joints. J. Anat. **66**, 210–227 (1932)

McCutchen, C.W.: A note upon tensile stress in the collagen fibers of articular cartilage. Med. Electron. Biol. Engn. **3**, 447–448 (1965)

McCutchen, C.W.: Boundary lubrication by synovial fluid: demonstration and possible osmotic explanation. Fed. Proc. **25**, 1061–1068 (1966)

McMurray, T.P.: Internal derangements of the knee joint. Ann. R. Coll. Surg. Engl. **3**, 210–219 (1948)

Meachim, G., Ghadially, F.N., Collins, D.H.: Regressive changes in the superficial layer of human articular cartilage. Ann. Rheum. Dis. **24**, 23–30 (1965)

Michaelis, L.: Kontrastfüllung des Kniegelenks mit Uroselektan. Röntgenpraxis **3**, 320–325 (1931)

Mittler, S., Freiberger, R.H., Harrison-Stubbs, M.: A method of improving cruciate ligament visualisation in double contrast arthrography. Radiology **102**, 441–442 (1972)

Müller, W.: Biologie der Gelenke. Leipzig: Barth 1929

Muir, H., Bullough, P., Maroudas, A.: The distribution of collagen in human articular cartilage with some of its physiological implications. J. Bone Joint Surg. **52B**, 554–563 (1970)

Nicholas, J.A., Freiberger, R.H., Killoran, P.J.: Double-contrast arthrography of the knee. Its value in the management of two hundred and twenty-five knee derangements. J. Bone Joint Surg. **52-A**, 203–220 (1970)

Olsen, R.W.: Knee arthrography. Am. J. Roentgenol. **101**, 897–914 (1967)

Outerbridge, R.E.: The etiology of chondromalacia patellae. J. Bone Joint Surg. **43-B**, 752–757 (1961)

Paul, J.P.: Bioengineering studies of the forces transmitted by joints. In: Biomechanics and related bioengineering topics. Kenedi, R.H. (ed.), p. 369–386. Oxford: Pergamon Press 1965

Pavlov, H., Freiberger, R., Deck, M.F., Morrissey, J.K.: Computer assisted tomography of the knee. RSNA scientific exhibition 1977

Radin, E.L., Bryan, R.S.: The effect of weight-bearing on regrowth of the medial meniscus after meniscectomy. J. Trauma **10**, 169–175 (1970)

Ricklin, P., Rüttimann, A., Del Buono, M.S.: Die Meniscusläsion. Stuttgart: Thieme 1964

Ricklin, P., Rüttimann, A., Del Buono, M.S.: Meniscus Lesions. Practical Problems of Clinical Diagnosis, Arthrography and Therapy. New York: Grune and Stratton 1971

Rijnks, J.: Chondropathia patellae. Groningen: Thesis 1976
Robinson, I., Werndorff, R.: Über die Sauerstoffinsufflation der Gelenke und Weichteile zu radiologisch-diagnostischen Zwecken. Arch. Phys. Med. u. med. Techn. **1**, 22–35 (1905/1906)
Roebuck, E.J.: Double contrast knee arthrography some new points of technique including the use of Dimer X. Clin. Radiol. **28**, 247–257 (1977)
Romaniuk, P.A., Thomas, G.: Der diagnostische Wert der Arthrographie bei Erkrankungen des Kniegelenkes. Radiol. Diagn. **9**, 516–527 (1968)
Salter, R.B., McNeil, R.: Pathological changes in articular cartilage secondary to persistent joint deformity. J. Bone Joint Surg. **47B**, 185–186 (1965)
Savastano, A.A., Poirier, P.E., Izzi, J.A.: Double contrast arthrography of the knee. A report of 135 consecutive studies at Rhode Island Hospital. Rhode Island Med. J. **56**, 423–426 (1974)
Shrive, N.: The weight-bearing role of the meniscus of the knee. J. Bone Joint Surg. **56B/2**, 381–386 (1974)
Smillie, J.S.: Observations on the regeneration of the semilunar cartilages in man. Br. J. Surg. **31**, 398–401 (1944)
Smillie, J.S.: Injuries of the knee joint. Edinburgh: Livingstone 1951
Smillie, J.S.: Diseases of the knee joint. Edinburgh: Livingstone 1974
Smillie, J.S.: Injuries of the knee. Ed. 4, Edinburgh: Livingstone (1975)
Sokoloff, L.: Elasticity of ageing cartilage. Fed. Proc. **25**, 1089–1095 (1966)
Sood, S.C.: A study of the effects of experimental immobilisation on rabbit articular cartilage. J. Anat. **108**, 497–507 (1971)
Spalteholz, W.: Handatlas und Lehrbuch der Anatomie des Menschen. Zürich, Stuttgart: Hirzel 1954
Staple, T.W.: Extrameniscal lesions demonstrated by double-contrast arthrography of the knee. Radiology **102**, 311–319 (1972)
Thiemann, W., Fischer, J.: Die postoperative arthrografische Beurteilung von Meniskusresten und Meniskusregeneraten. Fortschritte Röntgenstr. **112**, 759–767 (1970)
Thijn, C.J.P.: De correlatie tussen klinische en arthrografische bevindingen bij meniscusletsels. Ned. T. Geneesk. **112**, 1625–1630 (1968)
Thijn, C.J.P.: Dubbelcontrastarthrografie bij degeneratieve meniscusafwijkingen. Ned. T. Geneesk. **115**, 604–606 (1971)
Thijn, C.J.P.: Arthrography in lesions of both menisci in one knee joint. Arch. Chir. Neerl. **26/2**, 147–155 (1974)
Thijn, C.J.P.: Het Röntgenonderzoek van de knie. Ned. T. Geneesk. **119**, 1893–1899 (1975)
Thijn, C.J.P.: Double contrast arthrography in meniscal lesions and patellar chondropathy. Radiol. Clin. **45**, 345–362 (1976)
Trueta, J., Harrison, M.H.M.: Osteoarthritis of the hip: A study of the nature and evolution of the disease. J. Bone Joint Surg. **35B**, 442–461 (1953)
Uebermuth, H.: Meniskusexstirpation; Regeneration und Arthrosis deformans. Chirurg **13**, 329–334 (1941)
Van De Berg, F., Crèvecoeur, M.: Etude anatomique et radiologique du genou arthrographie. J. Belge Radiol. **34**, 7–82 (1951)
Van De Berg,F. Crèvecoeur, M.: La meniscographie en serie du genou. Acta Orthop. Belg. **19**, 293–306 (1953)

Van De Berg, F., Crèvecoeur, M.: La meniscographie en serie du genou (après 1000 examens). J. Radiol. Electrol. **36**, 389 (1955)
Walker, P.S.: The role of the menisci in force transmission across the knee. Clin. Orthop. No. **109**, 184–192 (1975)
Walker, P.S., Hajek, J.V.: The load-bearing area in the knee joint. J. Biomech. **5**, 581–589 (1972)
Wiberg, G.: Roentgenography and anatomic studies of the patello-femoral joint with special reference to chondromalacia patellae. Acta Orthop. Scand. **12**, 319–410 (1941)
Wiener, S.N.: Contrast arthrography of the knee joint: A comparison of positive and negative methods. Radiology **89**, 1083–1086 (1967)
Wilson, P.D., Eyre-Brook, A.L., Francis, J.D.: A clinical and anatomical study of the semimembranosus bursa in relation to popliteal cyst. J. Bone Joint Surg. **20**, 963–984 (1938)
Wolfe, R.D., Colloff, B.: Popliteal cysts. J. Bone Joint Surg. **54A**, 1057–1063 (1972)

Subject Index

Accuracy arthrography – arthroscopy
–, lateral meniscal lesions 59
–, medial meniscal lesions 56
–, patellar chondropathy 93, 94, 95
–, ruptures cruciate ligaments 117, 118
Accuracy arthrography – arthrotomy 2, 59, 60
Aftercare arthrography 10
Air embolism 1, 12
Allergic reactions 12
Anterior cruciate ligament
–, accuracy arthrography – arthroscopy 117, 118
–, anatomy 13, 97–100
–, etiology rupture 107
–, radiologic anatomy 102, 106
–, radiology rupture 110, 112, 113
Arthrography, technique 6–10
Arthroscopy; see also Accuracy
–, lateral meniscal lesions 32, 59
–, medial meniscal lesions 32, 55–57
–, patellar chondropathy 93, 94, 95
–, ruptures cruciate ligaments 117, 118
Arthrosis deformans 135, 138–141
Arthrotomy 60, 85
Articular cartilage
–, degeneration 3, 52, 66, 132, 135
–, histology 64, 135
–, lubrication 16–18
–, nutrition 65, 85, 140

Baker cyst 131–133, 140
Baumgartl dysplasia 75, 76, 78
Blumensaat line 82
Bucket – handle rupture 36

Capsule 119–126
Chondrocalcinosis 141
Collateral ligaments
–, anatomy 119, 126
–, ruptures 20, 54, 107, 137, 140
Combined meniscal rupture 36, 41
Complications arthrography 1, 10, 12
Computerized axial tomography
–, cruciate ligaments 102
–, patellofemoral joint 67
Contrast media 1, 5, 11, 12
Corpora libera 31, 34
Correlation arthrography – arthroscopy; see Accuracy
Cruciate ligaments; see also Anterior – and posterior cruciate ligament
–, anatomy 97–100
–, photography 6, 100, 102
–, ruptures 20, 54, 109, 132, 140
Cystic degeneration 20, 46, 48, 50

Degeneration articular cartilage 3, 52, 66, 132, 135
Degeneration meniscal cartilage 32, 40, 46, 50, 52, 54
Degeneration patellar cartilage 65, 72–75; see also Patellar chondropathy
Discoid meniscus 19, 43–46
Drawer sign 102, 116

Facies patellaris femoris
–, dysplasia 78–81, 136
Fish mouth rupture 36, 40, 41
Flaccid collateral ligaments 20, 25, 32, 102, 113
Foam, intra-articular 5, 31
Focus X-ray tube 6

Ganglion, see cystic degeneration
Gastrocnemial bursa 128; see also semimembranosogastrocnemial bursa

Hemarthros 85
Hemophilia 85, 140
High patella 82, 85
History of arthrography 1, 2
Hoffa body 21, 31, 40, 64, 105, 119–121
Hydrops 11, 85, 102, 124, 132

Immobilization of the knee joint 85
Infrapatellar synovial fold 21, 31, 64, 105

Intercondylar luxation in meniscal lesions 36

Lateral meniscus
–, accuracy arthrography – arthroscopy 59
–, anatomy 15
–, cystic degeneration 20, 46, 48, 50
–, discoid lateral meniscus 43–46
–, etiology of lesion 19, 20
–, mobility 18, 19
–, radiologic anatomy 25–27
–, technique of photography 6–8
Linea eminens 62, 72, 83, 89
Longitudinal rupture 33, 36, 37, 40, 57, 60
Low patella 83
Lubrication of the knee joint 16–18
Luxation of the patella; see subluxation

Measurements facies patellaris femoris 79
Measurements patella 77
Medial meniscus
–, accuracy arthrography – arthroscopy 56
–, anatomy 13, 97
–, etiology of lesion 18–20
–, mobility 18, 19
–, radiologic anatomy 20–25
–, regenerate 52, 138
–, technique photography 6–8
Meniscal remnant 52, 54, 142
Meniscectomy 16, 52, 72, 89, 91, 138
Meniscus
–, anatomy 13–15
–, central margin 8, 25, 40, 41, 57
–, degeneration, cystic 20, 46, 48, 50
–, degeneration, superficial 32, 40, 46, 50, 52, 54
–, degeneration, secondary 50, 52, 54
–, discoid meniscus 19, 43–46
–, etiology of lesion 18, 19, 20, 50
–, function 16
–, mobility 18, 19
–, radiologic anatomy 20–27
–, regenerate 52, 140
–, ruptures 32–42, 132, 136
– –, combined rupture 41
– –, fish mouth rupture 36, 40, 41
– –, longitudinal rupture 33, 36, 37, 40, 57, 60
– –, tangential incisure 18, 21, 32, 36, 47, 59
– –, transverse rupture 19, 40
–, technique of photography 6–8
Mucopolysaccharides 64, 66
Mucous ligament 21, 31, 64, 105

Negative contrast arthrography 1, 3

Osteochondritis dissecans 140

Patella
–, infera; see low patella
–, measurements 77
–, mobility increased 82, 83
–, partita 69, 78
–, tilting 84, 85, 89
Patellar cartilage; see articular cartilage
Patellar cartilage degeneration; see patellar chondropathy
Patellar chondropathy 3, 66, 67, 72, 75, 78, 82–95, 132
Patellar dysplasia 75, 77, 78, 85, 136
Patellofemoral joint 61, 67, 82, 85, 136
–, arthrosis 84, 89, 141
–, technique of photography 9, 89, 120
–, measurements 79
Popliteal bursa 27, 134
Popliteus muscle 15, 19, 26, 27, 106
Positive contrast arthrography 1, 3, 100
Posterior cruciate ligament
–, accuracy arthrography – arthroscopy 117, 118
–, anatomy 97–100
–, etiology of rupture 107, 108
–, radiologic anatomy 107, 108
–, radiology rupture 109, 112, 116
Posttraumatic dystrophy 85

Recess of the articular cavity 20, 21, 32
Regenerate 52, 138
Retinaculum patellae 63, 64, 85, 119
Rheumatoid arthritis 85, 122–124, 132, 133, 140

Schublade; see drawer sign
Secondary meniscal degeneration 50, 52, 54
Semimembranosogastrocnemial bursa 25, 128–132
Semimembranous bursa 128, 130; see also semimembranosogastrocnemial bursa
Spurious meniscal lesions 27, 31, 119
Subluxation of the patella 78, 82–85, 88, 89
Suprapatellar bursa 119, 127
Synovia 4, 16, 18

Synovial biopsy 11, 56
Synovial membrane 99, 100, 106, 119, 123, 124
Synovial hypertrophy 21, 32, 40
Synovitis 11, 123, 140

Tangential incisure 18, 21, 32, 36, 47, 59
Technique double contrast arthrography 3–10
Tilting patella 84, 85, 89
Transverse rupture 19, 40

Uratic arthritis 141
Urticaria 12

Wiberg III patella 75–78

Xerography
–, Baker cyst 120
–, chronic synovitis 122
–, cruciate ligaments 102
–, Hoffa body 120

Advances in Artificial Hip and Knee Joint Technology

Editors: M. Schaldach, D. Hohmann
In collaboration with R. Thull, F. Hein

1976. 525 figures. XII, 525 pages
(Engineering in Medicine, Vol. 2)
ISBN 3-540-07728-6

H.-R. Henche

Die Arthroskopie des Kniegelenks

Mit einem Geleitwort von E. Morscher

1978. 163. Abbildungen, davon 66 farbig,
1 Tabelle. X, 86 Seiten
ISBN 3-540-08380-4
Arthroscopy of the Knee, English Edition due for publication in Summer 1979

Late Reconstructions of Injured Ligaments of the Knee

Editors: K.-P. Schulitz, H. Krahl, W.H. Stein
With contributions by M.E. Blazina, D.H. O'Donoghue, S.L. James, J.C. Kennedy, A. Trillat

1978. 42 figures, 21 tables. V, 120 pages
ISBN 3-540-08720-6

P.G.J. Maquet

Biomechanics of the Knee

With Application to the Pathogenesis and the Surgical Treatment of Osteoarthritis

1976. 184 figures. XIII, 230 pages
ISBN 3-540-07882-7

M. Watanabe, S. Takeda, H. Ikeuchi

Atlas of Arthroscopy

3rd edition 1979. 226 figures. X, 156 pages
Igaku Shoin Ltd., Tokyo
ISBN 3-540-07674-3
Distribution rights for USA, Canada and Europe: Springer-Verlag

Progress in Orthopaedic Surgery

Editorial Board: N. Gschwend, D. Hohmann, J.L. Hughes, D.S. Hungerford, G.D. MacEwen, E. Morscher, J. Schatzker, H. Wagner, U.H. Weil

Volume 1

Leg Length Discrepancy The Injured Knee

Editor: D.S. Hungerford
With contributions by numerous experts

1977. 100 figures. X, 160 pages
ISBN 3-540-08037-6

Volume 3

The Knee: Ligament and Articular Cartilage Injuries

Guesteditor: D.E. Hastings
With contributions by numerous experts

1978. 139 figures, 20 tables. X, 191 pages
ISBN 3-540-08679-X

Related Journals:

Skeletal Radiology

International Orthopaedics

Archives of Orthopaedic and Traumatic Surgery / Archiv für orthopädische und Unfall-Chirurgie

Springer-Verlag
Berlin
Heidelberg
New York

Springer AV Instruction Program

Films:

Theoretical and practical bases of internal fixation, results of experimental research:

Internal Fixation – Basic Principles and Modern Means

The Biomechanics of Internal Fixation

The Ligaments of the Knee Joint Pathophysiology

Internal fixation of fractures and in corrective surgery:

Internal Fixation of Forearm Fractures

Internal Fixation of Noninfected Diaphyseal Pseudarthroses

Internal Fixation of Malleolar Fractures

Internal Fixation of Patella Fractures

Medullary Nailing

Internal Fixation of the Distal End of the Humerus

Internal Fixation of Mandibular Fractures

Corrective Osteotomy of the Distal Tibia

Internal Fixation of Tibial Head Fractures
(available in German only)

Joint replacement:

Total Hip Prostheses (3 parts)
Part 1: Instruments. Operation on Model
Part 2: Operative Technique
Part 3: Complications. Special Cases

Elbow-Arthroplasty with the New GSB-Prosthesis

Total Wrist Joint Replacement

Slide Series:

ASIF-Technique for Internal Fixation of Fractures

Manual of Internal Fixation
(in preparation)

The Ligaments of Knee Joint – Pathophysiology
(in preparation)

Small Fragment Set Manual

Internal Fixation of Patella and Malleolar Fractures

Total Hip Prostheses
Operation on Model and in vivo, Complications and Special Cases

Asepsis in Surgery

- Further films and slide series in preparation
- Technical data: 16 mm and super-8 (color, magnetic sound, optical sound), videocassettes. Slide series in ringbinders
- Films in English or German, several in French; slide series with multilingual legends
- Please ask for information material

Sales:
Springer-Verlag,
Heidelberger Platz 3,
D-1000 Berlin 33,

or

Springer-Verlag New York Inc
175 Fifth Avenue,
New York, NY 10010

Springer-Verlag
Berlin
Heidelberg
New York

MIX
Papier aus verantwortungsvollen Quellen
Paper from responsible sources
FSC® C105338

If you have any concerns about our products,
you can contact us on
ProductSafety@springernature.com

In case Publisher is established outside the EU,
the EU authorized representative is:
Springer Nature Customer Service Center GmbH
Europaplatz 3, 69115 Heidelberg, Germany

Printed by Libri Plureos GmbH
in Hamburg, Germany